Praise for Understand and Overcome Your Chronic Pain

"A more comprehensive and useful guide to pain will be hard to find – it is wise, informative, and very practical. And then there's the empathy and compassion that runs through every page. It will be an eye-opener for sufferers and practitioners alike."

Stephen Rollnick, PhD
Honorary Distinguished Professor,
School of Medicine, Cardiff University

"Richmond Stace's book Understand and Overcome Your Chronic Pain *is a really important self-help book for those suffering from long-term pain. The golden message is that with education and help you can modify and alleviate your pain; it is not what is done to you but what you can do for yourself that makes the difference. The understanding of pain and its management has changed radically over the last two decades during which Richmond has been at the leading edge of these ideas and has incorporated them into his practise for the betterment of his patients. This book will give the person suffering from long-term pain, hope and strategies for alleviation of their suffering and is much to be recommended."*

J Richard Smith MB ChB, MD, FRCOG
Professor of Practice, Consultant Gynaecological Surgeon,
Imperial College, London, UK
Hon Consultant in Transplantation Surgery, Oxford
University Hospitals, Oxford, UK

"We'll definitely be stocking it, and I'll be recommending the heck out of it. I wasn't sure what to expect, but your holistic approach is encapsulated by this brilliant book. I found it quite moving as well as helpful. In modern speak, I felt 'seen'."

Christian Haddow Butcher
Bookseller, Daunt Books

*"*Understand and Overcome Your Chronic Pain *by Richmond Stance is the most amazing, thoughtful, and honest book. Combining his experience in the clinic with his powerful knowledge from different fields, Richmond created a special gift for anyone who is experiencing chronic pain, friends and family who want to help, and healthcare providers. The unique approach of revealing methods that really work will plant the*

seeds of confidence that everything is possible once again, even living with chronic pain. It is a very powerful gem of a book."

Anca M.

"When Richmond first told me he was writing a book I was very excited, I absolutely love the content he shares on his social media, so I had a feeling that any book he wrote about overcoming chronic pain would become a 'must-read'.

I was right!

As the book unfolds, it becomes clear that this is different from every other book on pain that's out there, as great as they are.

Richmond's introduction is great, it tells the reader who he is and where he's coming from, it makes you feel like he's got a reassuring arm around your shoulder as you embark on the journey together, because chronic pain management is too often a lonely place to be!

A great line that jumped out at me was 'Now is that moment because this is the only moment'. Many of us with chronic pain spend so much striving to get back to the person we were and longing for the day in the future when our pain will be gone, instead of focusing on what we CAN do right now!

The book is sprinkled throughout with 'Encouragement Points' which I found extremely useful to easily summarise what I'd read.

This book gives people a completely different lens through which they can look at pain. Whether a healthcare practitioner or a person living with pain or even someone supporting a friend or relative with pain, I can't recommend this book enough. You will want to devour it whole in one sitting and keep it with you as you change direction and choose a different path to overcome/live well with your pain!

I predict this being a No. 1 Bestseller."

Louise Trewern
National Pain Advocate
Fellow Durham University Wolfson Research
Institute for Health & Wellbeing Lead Lived
Experience Trainer Live Well With Pain
Immediate Past Vice Chair British Pain
Society Patient Voice Committee

"It is going to be amazing! I am very excited to see it published as I like it a lot!

Reading your first draft was just at the perfect time as I came out of my pain hangover, and it has helped me get myself out of the darkness. So thank you … although you had no idea you were helping me of course!

As a person who lives, I mean really lives, alongside my pain, I'm always looking for hope when reading about pain. Richmond, as I totally expected, your book is brimming with much-needed gentleness and hope for people like me in pain. Without hope, I often find that pain can consume my life, but with hard work life can instead consume the pain. I was having a look at the definitions of hope, and it was interesting to see that an archaic definition of hope is trust. Interestingly, it is this aspect of hope that brings me life: trust in my own abilities to live with pain. Your writing feels very trustworthy. My yoga head cries out, this book is a safe space.

Your writing guides the reader compassionately. This style is like a friend to accompany me in my pain. When pain becomes lonely a good trusty friend is much appreciated, in any form.

The Encouragement Points are just so spot on and perfect idea for this kind of book."

Ruth Barber

"Understand and Overcome Your Chronic Pain *is a must-read for everyone, as we will all experience pain throughout our life. But for those with chronic pain, Richmond's book is a beacon of hope that things can and do get better. It is a testament to his dedication to reaching and helping as many people as possible. In* Understand and Overcome Your Chronic Pain, *Richmond Stace extends his healing touch to a broader audience, and I have no doubt that it will be a source of empowerment and transformation for many. This book is not just a must-read, it is a must-apply guide for reclaiming a life free from the burdens of chronic pain.*

I have had the privilege of being Richmond's patient and have witnessed firsthand his remarkable expertise in the field of chronic pain management. Richmond's work is nothing short of transformative. His approach goes beyond conventional methods, equipping individuals with a toolbox of practical strategies to navigate and conquer chronic pain. Through his guidance, I have gained invaluable insights and skills that have empowered me to take control of my pain and enhance my overall well-being. What sets Richmond apart is his unwavering commitment to making a tangible difference in the lives of those grappling with chronic pain. His book, based on his day-to-day work, reflects this commitment. It is a treasure trove of knowledge and practical offerings providing readers a wealth of techniques that can be immediately integrated into their lives."

Dr Jennifer Ellen Hamer

"Richmond Stace has transformed how I view pain (as a doctor), and he has helped so many of my patients find their way through dark times. Not infrequently they had been dismissed or sometimes even abandoned by clinicians, who couldn't explain or 'fix' their pain.

This book teaches a person how they can gain control of their pain, by first understanding it and then using learned skills to live a desired life, rather than 'waiting to get better', first.

If you're suffering in pain, or if you work with patients who are experiencing pain, this book will be your very best educator, journey companion, and encourager. I urge you to read it and be enlightened."

Dr Cath Spencer-Smith
Sports Medicine Consultant

Understand and Overcome Your Chronic Pain

Understand and Overcome Your Chronic Pain

The Comprehensive Guide to
Chronic Pain and How You Can Shape
a Positive Future

Richmond Stace

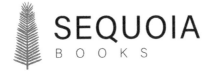

SEQUOIA
B O O K S

First published in 2023 by Sequoia Books

ISBN
Print: 9781914110283
EPUB: 9781914110290

A CIP record for this book is available from the British Library

Library of Congress Cataloguing-In-Publication Data

Name: Richmond Stace
Title: Understand and Overcome Your Chronic Pain/Stace
Description: 1st Edition, Sequoia Books UK 2023
Print: 9781914110283
EPUB: 9781914110290

Library of Congress Control Number: 2023919589

Print and Electronic production managed by Deanta Global

Contents

Acknowledgements

Thanks to:

The people on this journey with me: Jo, Lucy, Sam, Rosie, Poppy.

My mentors who have shaped my way of being, in particular Mike Pegg (The Encourager) and Mick Thacker.

Major influencers on my on-going work, including Mark Miller, Andy Clark, Anil Seth, Anna Ciaunica, Professor Stephen Rollnick and Jeff Weigh.

And very importantly, giving me purpose, all the people I have had the privilege to help and care for.

Section 1 Introduction

Contents

Forewords by Mike Pegg and Dr Mark Miller

Foreword: Mike Pegg

There are many ways to live life. One approach is to pass on knowledge that people can use in their daily lives and work. Richmond is somebody who takes this path. He aims to encourage, educate, and enable people to shape a positive future.

Great educators often focus on inspiration, implementation, and integration. They aim (a) to create an inspiring environment, (b) to provide practical tools that work, and (c) to enable people to integrate the learning in their own way.

This is an approach that Richmond follows in his practice and in this book. Like many fine educators, he shares knowledge in ways that are personal, practical, and, in the widest sense, profitable.

Personal—it should relate to the person's goals;
Practical—it should provide practical tools that work;
Profitable—it should help the person to achieve their goals.

Great educators often embody the qualities demonstrated by sages. They also realise, however, that they will always be lifetime students. This means they will be continually learning and trying to improve.

Richmond's work embodies many of these qualities. Plus, most of all, a generosity of spirit. As ever, he wants to pass on knowledge that works. You will, of course, use these ideas in your own way to shape a positive future.

Foreword: Dr Mark Miller

In the world of healthcare, where the challenges are as diverse as the individuals seeking help, there exists a guiding light—a compassionate, experienced professional who has dedicated nearly three decades of his life to aiding others in their journey towards better health. *Understand and Overcome Your Chronic Pain: The Comprehensive Guide to Chronic Pain and How You Can Shape a Positive Future* represents the culmination of Richmond Stace's immense experience and knowledge, offering a fresh perspective on pain management that challenges conventional paradigms.

The heart of this book beats with empathy for those grappling with pain and suffering. While Richmond acknowledges that the path to recovery is anything but easy, he firmly believes that it is possible. Drawing on the latest scientific insights into pain, he proposes a new paradigm—one rooted in the individual's strengths, potential and ability to shape a positive future. The reader is encouraged to see pain not as an insurmountable obstacle but as an experience that can be managed, even transformed, by understanding its underlying mechanisms and learning essential life skills.

This book is a beacon of hope for those navigating the complex world of chronic pain. It encourages readers to harness their strengths, embrace their positive history of overcoming challenges and develop essential life skills. It emphasizes that overcoming pain is not a solitary journey but a collaborative effort, offering guidance and support to individuals, therapists and clinicians alike. In many ways, *Understand and Overcome Your Chronic Pain* is not so much a book as a compassionate companion on the path towards a better life.

A note from me

I wish you a warm welcome.

I have had the privilege of working in healthcare since 1993 when I started my training as a registered nurse. Not far off 30 years of being a professional helper, albeit with different hats.

In this time, I have spent time with thousands of people who have found themselves in challenging positions with their health. From the outset every action has been about helping the person in front of me, however I can, to improve their life. This is how I was trained. I am truly grateful for that training and the people who taught and influenced me.

In this brief note, I simply want to say that having spent all this time with so many people, I know that dealing with pain and suffering is one of, if not the, hardest thing for a human to have to do. As I write about all the different things you can do, at no time do I believe that this is easy. It can get *easier*, but it is not easy. But I also know you can do it.

You can use your strengths and abilities to understand yourself, your pain, and what you can do to achieve freedom in your life.

Freedom from suffering is possible when you are open to life and what it offers. The fact that you are currently struggling is not an indication of how it needs to be moving forwards. It is also not your fault. You did not choose to be in this situation, or even to be you with your embodied mind. But now you can choose a better way forward with the intention of overcoming your pain and living your best life. Your intentions, your beliefs, your expectations, and actions shape your way forwards, starting now.

Pain may not be what you think it is as you will discover. You know what your pain feels like for sure (the experience), but the things that shape your pain could be new to you. Further, understanding and knowing how you can control these influential factors will empower and enable you. You will be able to let go of limiting beliefs and avoidances, by reconnecting with what matters, as you will see when you read this book. I am excited to share this with you.

I have the greatest respect for your efforts and what you have and are trying to do to make a better life. It takes courage, determination, and perseverance. You are showing all of these. You are doing your best.

With that in mind, I hope you find what I have to say helpful, useful, and meaningful, despite the fact that it may be difficult. There are perhaps new concepts, facts about pain and ways to move forward that challenge your existing beliefs. I know that, because of the daily conversations I have with people who are suffering.

I want you to know that each word I write comes through the lens of a caring concern for you that I hope will translate into action that shapes a positive future for you.

You can overcome.

A premise

There is a premise upon which the book is based, which I describe for you here. Some of the points may appear to be obvious, but they bring clarity to my messages and approach to helping you from the outset.

There will be some information that you may be familiar with and some new. The traditional paradigm for treating pain is not working, which is why chronic pain is one of the largest global health burdens. In this book, I present to you a different paradigm that is based on the latest science and understanding of pain and related fields. Some of this may sound and feel quite different. In some ways, I hope that it does. If you are struggling with your pain despite your best efforts, you may need other knowledge and skills to get unstuck and move forward.

My intent is to guide and encourage you alongside what you are already doing, some of which may be with a therapist or clinician.

This will begin to set the scene and be clarified as you read on.

A couple of important terms to clarify: The positive approach and overcoming pain

'Overcoming pain is something that you do, not something that is done to you'

The title of the book talks of a positive approach and overcoming pain. I think that it is important to clarify what I mean.

The positive approach is not the same as positive thinking, which can be saying all is well when it is not. Instead, the positive approach is about clarifying your picture of success and taking steps each day in that direction. There is a focus on your strengths and potential to shape a positive future.

The notion of overcoming pain is a personal one, depending on your circumstances—you should always consider the circumstances because this is what helps establish an accurate view of the situation. This is an important part of the initial thinking and conversation in a programme. You want to aim for the best and realistic outcomes. So what does overcoming pain mean?

For some people, this will be a complete easing of the particular pain of concern. Having said that, it is important to realise that once you have had significant pain, it is more likely that you will feel it again at some point in the future. Not because there is an actual problem, but due to something similar in the present circumstances as it was before.

Knowing this is important because you can manage that moment skilfully and compassionately rather than worry, you have somehow re-injured yourself or that the pain is back for good. This demonstrates the power of your thinking and beliefs about your pain, as they determine what you tell yourself and do, actually shaping what is to come. The same is true the other way around, meaning that if you truly understand pain, you will navigate yourself towards getting better.

For many people, overcoming pain means that pain is no longer the predominant force in their life. They are free from prolonged suffering. There are moments of pain, but they also know that they experience other perceptions—there are many of these. With a focus on living your best life, including daily skills of being well, you learn how to ease your suffering (a skill you can develop with practice) when needed and to fully immerse in joyful and pleasurable activities as they happen.

To do this means you must learn to be present and see the difference between what is really occurring and what you are telling yourself. This is a skill, making an enormous difference in how you self-rate your progress. You may think you are doing worse than you really are when the focus is on the tough times, rather than the bigger picture when you notice other moments of joy and pleasure, usefulness, and contribution. Learning how to create these situations is another practice and skill, as you will see.

Much of our experience depends on what we expect to happen, based on what has happened before. From that though, I hope you can see the opportunity to actively shape something better. This is the purpose of the book of course.

It is the case that when certain conditions feature pain, overcoming pain would mean that the person is living life in the best way that they can, trying to focus on what is possible: What can I do and build upon? Medical treatment can be useful and important, but life skills are what brings the quality, and are available to everyone. The approach you take, the attitude, and the effort are things you can control. Together with the modern understanding of pain, this brings great hope.

Overcoming pain essentially means making a better life in the many ways in which you can. I believe that whatever the start point, you can improve your life, and that there are many ways you can do this practically. This is my encouragement to you. With everyone I work with, I expect them to improve their lives in many ways, particularly when they free themselves from limiting beliefs and perceived inadequacies.

You have strengths. You have a positive history of dealing with and overcoming challenges. You have these resources and can access them now.

Now is the time to create a new story and new experiences for yourself.

Some key points to consider

1. You are experiencing persistent pain (also known as chronic pain and on-going pain) and want to improve your life.
2. Pain is a whole person experience that is felt in your lived world.
3. Pain is what you say it is.
4. Pain is always real.
5. You can improve your life.
6. You will try some of the practices and use some of the tools in your own world. I do not expect you to simply believe what I say, but instead to have your own experiences as a basis for your faith in what you are doing.
7. Focus on what you want rather than what you don't want.
8. Think about what you can do and build, rather than what you cannot.
9. I want this to be a helpful and encouraging guide. It will not necessarily be for everyone, but I hope many benefit.
10. There is no single practice that works in isolation. Instead, it is about how you construct your own path forwards, working towards your picture of success. With encouragement and support.
11. I take a person-centred over body-centred approach, which I hope comes across strongly in this book.
12. You have strengths that you can use to overcome your pain.
13. You have a positive history of successes that you can use now to fortify your efforts and build upon.
14. You have skills already that you have been using, some of which will continue to be helpful.
15. This is a collaboration between you and the therapists and/or clinicians you work with, including me at a distance via these words.

Section 2 My journey into pain

When I left school in 1992, I didn't have many ideas for my future. Project 2000 Nursing was suggested. This was a university-based nurse training bringing more academia to the field. I thought that it sounded interesting and so I applied, which I think surprised a few people.

Offered a place, I took it up and found myself getting immersed in the world of healthcare. I was 19 and getting my first exposure to people's lives and suffering.

At school I was a reluctant and choosy learner, much preferring sport and other extracurricular activities. But now I was interested. I discovered a passion for pathophysiology and trying to match the science with people's experiences and presentations.

We had one particular tutor who was not only firm with us but also compassionate and showed great caring. His sessions were dedicated to understanding people's experiences through the lens of biology, but never forgetting the human being. Another gave us a lesson on how to shave a man's face, which has always stuck with me. Something simple, yet important to the person who cannot do this for himself. What must this be like, I wondered?

These and many other experiences started to open my eyes to the person-first approach, although I did not know it was called that at the time. I was still mostly into facts, wanting to understand how the body worked, what happens when it goes wrong, and what medicine or surgery had to offer in response. In other words, how to fix people.

Over the next three years, I spent my time seeing and doing as much as I could. I don't think there was a department I missed. Outside of the formal training, I worked as a nursing auxiliary (now called a Healthcare Assistant) on the wards, clocking up many hours, night and day.

The hands-on work was a superb learning experience. There was and is no better way to learn about human nature. In my opinion, all healthcare professionals should spend a year or so working on the wards before they embark on their chosen path.

At the end of the training, we had to produce a final project. I chose to look at how people recovered from operations, having noticed that the same procedure would often result in very different experiences for the patients. This was my second venture into understanding pain.

Prior to this, I had spent some time with the hospital pain team. We would visit people on the wards who had been referred for pain management. It was mostly about drugs, but I saw that spending time by listening to the person and being present had a good effect.

To be honest, I cannot recall what I discovered in my project. It may be sitting somewhere in a dusty cardboard box. But I do know that a seed was sown.

I remember because some years later I was sitting in a lecture about pain, it all came back. There was a sudden realisation, an explosion of thoughts and excitement. I had come full circle, back to the need to consider the whole person.

It was Mick Thacker who gave that lecture at St Thomas's, and I have not looked back since. What struck me was that there was known biology that could explain people's experiences of pain. But not just their pain, their overall state.

This was back in early 2000, and so much has changed since then. However, at the time, I knew that this was the path I wanted to pursue. I must admit, whilst a huge part of the feeling came from insights into how we can help people suffering persistent pain, I was also energised by the sense of rebellion against the existing outdated approaches. We could make a difference, help people, and move the field on in a positive direction. All held great appeal.

Recently I was told about Positive Deviance by Mike Pegg who has kindly written the introduction. These are 'uncommon behaviours and strategies' used by people to find better solutions (Positive Deviance Collaborative, positive-deviance.org). Mike puts it as behaving 'in ways that are different from others in their community. They experience similar circumstances but the strategies they follow provide solutions to challenges.' This resonates enormously, putting words to how I feel I approach helping people.

When Mick started the Pain: Science and Society MSc at Kings, I knew that this was my next step. Yes, you could say I was now addicted to learning, but this was purely because my purpose had become clear. This was my fourth outing at university—11 years in total. I was working throughout, so not just ivory towers!

The two years spent with Mick and my year group (a terrific bunch of clinicians from different fields and places) were transformative. It was not just about learning pain science but developing skills on how to question, scrutinise, debate, and present ideas. Coffee shop meetings round a table discussing papers each week were part of our routine, but so was checking in on each other. We were a team.

The importance of those two years was paramount. It gave perspective and was a launch pad for future work that I felt could make a significant impact.

The idea of working with people suffering chronic pain using the latest understanding of pain was formed early in the course. By the time I finished at King's College London, I had a clear route forward. I was going to specialise and really focus on helping the people who were stuck with their pain. From this emerged Specialist Pain Physio, the brand I created.

Until recently, this was the identity of my work. Now I am more 'me', which has evolved over time as I have shaped my approach to helping and guiding people.

My second great influence on the journey was Mike Pegg, the pioneer of strength-based coaching. I used to go to different types of conferences and meetings, realising that deepening one's understanding of pain was not just about the science of it. I needed to understand human beings and their behaviours. To do this meant listening to and reading work from many fields: for example, psychology, philosophy, advertising, and copywriting.

On this occasion, I was at a strength-coaching conference. The attendees were lawyers, human resources managers, business coaches, change consultants, CEOs, leaders, and others from the business world. When we had to introduce ourselves round my table, I said, 'I'm a physio'. There were inquisitive looks. Someone asked me why I was there. It had already become clear to me that although our industries were different, we actually faced similar problems that had similar solutions: people getting stuck and then what we can do to encourage them to move forward.

Mike Pegg gave a talk at that conference, taking us on a journey through his career, influence, and approach. Much like Mick's talk on pain, this was another big moment as I realised that this was a way that I could work with people suffering from chronic pain. In fact, part of me felt that I was already doing something like this.

After the talk, Mike was kind enough to have a chat, and a few weeks later we had a deeper chat on Skype. Since, Mike has played an enormous role in helping and guiding me to shape a way of helping people in my own way.

A third person I would like to mention is business coach Alan Wick. We were introduced and met for a coffee. Alan has told me many useful things, but one message has always stuck: sharpen your arrow. In other words, be absolutely clear on your message. What is so important about this? Put simply, the message you communicate is the one that you are giving to others and will guide what you do.

I am forever tinkering with words, messages, and the way I communicate about pain. This was a key learning for me, and I still continue to try and sharpen my arrow. Helping people understand their pain is such a vital and first step. The way we do this has to be clear and have meaning for the person. This is why we should continue to sharpen, review, and re-review our messages.

This was my journey into pain. Of course, this is a brief summary and many other things have happened along the way. But I hope it gives you a sense of why I do what I do now: bringing together the latest pain science, coaching, compassion, and all my experiences, with a human and person-focused approach to helping people forge better ways of living, to bring greater happiness and connection to what they do in their lives—your life.

This is the purpose of the book. To share with you my knowledge and wisdom in a practical way that will enable you to live your best life.

Section 3 Setting the scene

Contents

Introduction

Pain is an experience that we all share as humans, except in a few who have a rare genetic condition. A vital part of the way we learn and survive, pain is necessary and normal.

There is a message wrapped up and delivered personally and uniquely to the person who perceives the pain. This can be as simple as a gentle request to look after your body or as complex as persisting suffering that is scantily linked to the state of your flesh and blood, better linked to the state of you, the person in your lived world.

Philosophers have long discussed pain as an experience perceived by the individual. Centuries after the topic was first raised, scientists and clinicians took up the mantle. Most notably and to be considered the fathers of pain medicine and science were Ron Melzack and Pat Wall.

Melzack and Wall questioned the existing idea that a message was sent to the brain from the injured body resulting in pain. In this model, the brain was a passive recipient, which is in huge contrast to current thinking. Their early work emerged as the Gate Theory of Pain before Melzack went on to describe the pain matrix, a distributed network of neurons in the brain that when active underpin the pain experience. This was the basis for thinking 'pain is in the brain'. This message is still common, but an inaccurate view as you will discover. You are more than a brain, and pain is not 'in there'.

Arguably the most important feature of Melzack and Wall's thinking was that the brain and other parts of the nervous system could modulate signals. This meant that pain could and did vary according to circumstances.

A number of notable scientists picked up the baton and ran. Today we can be thankful for their work as now there is much hope, especially in understanding and helping people who suffer chronic (persistent) pain.

Chronic (persistent) pain is one of the largest global health burdens (GBD, 2016). It affects millions and costs billions (Societal Impact of Pain, 2017). The numbers are not improving either, with more recent figures highlighting an increase in the percentage of people in pain from 26.3 in 2009 to 32.1 in 2021 (Macchia, 2022).

Despite these numbers and the fact that pain is a common reason for seeking help, the amount of time spent educating healthcare professionals remains minimal. In many cases, clinicians will receive just a few hours to understand pain. And perhaps more significantly, the biomedical model that is proven to be inadequate and frequently a barrier to improving quality of life remains the predominant way. Imagine in another field of work a situation where you have a model that does not work, which continues to be used.

If people working in healthcare do not understand pain and the model does not work, how can we help the people who suffer?

The misunderstanding of pain is reflected in society. People are lucky if they are given the facts about their pain based on modern knowledge. Most receive explanations based on outdated concepts, many of which are wrong.

When a person goes to see their doctor or another healthcare professional, they want to know what is going on, what they can do about it themselves, what help is available, and some timelines. Part of this must be understanding their pain. Without this, fear can easily continue or build, which contributes to the pain itself or they can easily head down the wrong path.

Essentially, you want to feel that you are in control. Most, if not all, who come to see me with their chronic pain do not feel that they are in control. Also, any control that they did have was removed by passive treatments: for example, take a pill, lie down, and receive an intervention.

Whilst there can be a role for such methods, they must sit within an approach that gives you a way forward that is active—to get better is an active process. Only you the individual can do this, with support, encouragement, and guidance. Overall though, you feel more in control with both willpower and way-power.

This book is all about you gaining control. From understanding your pain to a range of practices, tools, exercises, and strategies, you will be equipped to make the best choices to shape your positive future: knowledge, skills, and know-how.

The focus is always upon you and what you want to achieve in your life. This is the biggest theme for overcoming pain—living life is the best pain reliever. You choose to live your life now in the best way that you can, considering the ever-changing circumstances, rather than wait for a special moment when you feel ready to start. Many people are waiting for this time, hoping that a treatment of some kind will allow them to begin.

My message to you is that now is that moment because this is the only moment. Future and past are imagined and in memory, respectively. They are not happening except in your (embodied) mind. Whilst the thoughts are real and convincing, they are stories about what is happening. But is the thought true or actually happening right now? Realising this is a powerful practice as you will see.

Living in your best way is closely linked with building wellness, our greatest buffer to life's inevitable ups and downs. In my experience, coming through a wellness lens and learning to live once more allows you to concentrate on deepening connections with, or reconnecting with what really matters in your life. This comes from letting go of limiting beliefs, tapping into your strengths, living your values, and seeing possibilities.

The traditional way of thinking about treating pain does not work. This is borne out in the statistics about chronic pain and people's experiences. Undoubtedly, healthcare professionals and others want to help, but the thinking is often wrong, based on the wrong model.

You may be surprised to read that I do not believe we can treat pain. Why? Because there is nothing concrete to actually treat. This is the old model that is known as biomedical, which is the search for a pathology or a structural reason for pain. This way of thinking is fundamentally flawed because pain is not produced by the body tissues.

Let me clarify this important point for you from the outset. The body tissues do not have the ability to produce pain. Whilst you do experience pain in your body, the pain is not being generated from the place where you feel it. Confused?

This is the same for all experiences including hunger. Hunger is not produced by your stomach, and thirst is not produced by your mouth. All these examples, as with all states we perceive, are whole-person. In other words, you are the one who experiences pain, hunger, and laughter, not the body parts. The modern term is 'the lived experience', which is what it is like for you.

Your lived experiences are generated top down by the ensemble of body systems that include the nervous system (brain, spinal cord, and peripheral nerves), the immune system, the endocrine system, and the autonomic nervous system (Kiverstein et al., 2022; Nave et al., 2022). The systems very much work together, fully integrated rather than the separateness you may imply from textbooks.

So, if we can't treat pain per se, what are we actually doing? Why is it that if you rub a sore area it feels better? Well, of course, it doesn't always get better and sometimes can make it worse. That is because you are not touching the pain itself (you can't because there is nothing to touch), instead you are trying to change your biological state by taking some action and hence change your experience.

In other words, you are not treating the pain, instead you are seeking to feel better by altering the way your body systems are generating the experience. Put another way, you are creating the conditions to feel better, which you can do in many ways as you will read and hopefully practice. As a clinician or therapist, this is the same. There is no fixing or treating. There are only ways to help you create the conditions for a better, healthier state and hence life, to emerge.

Further, the healthcare system very much focuses on deficits and problems to solve. Of course, this feels right because this is the system that you have grown up in. Surely when you are unwell, there is a problem that needs to be diagnosed and then treated? All very familiar. And yes of course, if there is a condition that requires medical intervention to create the conditions for you to become well again, this is wise action.

But you are not just a passenger on the ride. This is your life that you are living. You are the one who is getting better actively, by creating the right conditions. This includes seeking help, taking medication, receiving other medical interventions, and living the best way that you can using life skills and the skills of being well, considering the ever changing circumstances. In other words, life is dynamic with no moment ever being the same.

There is a problem with fixating on problems and deficits. By studying these, you keep them at the forefront, ensuring disempowerment and the sense that there is something wrong with you. There is nothing wrong with you. You are the one experiencing the pain, the anxiety, the condition. You are not the pain, the anxiety, the condition. You do not need fixing.

Instead, you can study what goes well in your life and when you are at your best and healthiest. What are you thinking? What are you doing? How do you embody these states? By modelling these and getting into such states, you are building wellness and living.

There is a simple life rule. Focus on what you want rather than what you don't want. What do you want? Usually, a happy and healthy life. When have you been happy in your life? Even thinking about it can change the way you feel now. Try it if you like. Sit up a little straighter, close your eyes, and think of a specific time when you were really happy. What was happening for you? What was your facial expression? Where were you? Build the image and immerse yourself in it. Notice how you feel now.

Studying your successful styles when you were in flow and when you overcame challenges gives you a positive way forward. You can build on these and develop your skills plus learn others to work towards your picture of success.

I hope that this sounds different from your existing approach. It may even feel rather uncomfortable because of your current way of thinking about your situation. But there is the opportunity and the work to be done. Any time you feel uncomfortable, anxious, worried, frustrated, irritated, angry, life is revealing where you need to go to transform yourself and hence your life. This is available to you now and the purpose of my work. To help you achieve freedom.

In principle, to understand and overcome pain is simple. You update your knowledge, eliminate your fears, use your resilience, strengths, and positive history, and work towards your pictures of success. Easy right? No, not usually. Why? Because you are human and complex and have a tricky mind. We all do! Limiting beliefs, existing world views, and wrong thinking all take you down the wrong path, often underestimating your potential. Add the wrong messages from society and the healthcare system, it becomes even more confusing.

But this need not be the case. You can choose your approach and here I offer you one based on the latest thinking in pain and human potential.

My hope is that this book makes a useful and positive contribution to your life in a practical way. I conceived the Pain Coaching approach as a way of helping people understand their pain and to move on to live fulfilling lives. Day to day I work with people in the clinic and online, making sense of their pain, reducing fear, and then designing a way forward so that they feel free to live their best life. The individual is encouraged and guided onwards not only using the tools and practices but also having the all-important know-how to achieve their best results. With this book and these words, I hope to encourage you too.

Whilst a book does not replace face-to-face human connection and touch, the aim is that you use the Pain Coach approach in your own way, building on your strengths and things that truly work for you. This can be alongside existing treatment(s), rehabilitation, and therapy, as pain-coaching is designed to work with other therapies.

With that, I wish you the best with your onward journal as you take control and move on to a healthier and happier life.

'Happiness is not something ready made. It comes from your own actions.' The Dalia Lama

Who is this book for?

If you have picked it up, it's probably for you. But just in case you're not sure, I am writing for people suffering persistent or chronic pain in whatever form it takes—there are many. Whilst there is usually a musculoskeletal aspect for many, narrowing our thinking down to a body system moves away from the truth. Most people who I work with have more than one painful experience.

Often there are a range of pains such as headache, migraine, jaw pain, stomach pain, and pelvic pain together with the reason for coming along. Anxiety, depression, loneliness, post-traumatic stress disorder (PTSD), low self-worth, a strong self-critic, perfectionism, low expectations, and limiting beliefs are common. Of course, these feelings and experiences come as one rather than separately. You only have one unified experience, which is embodied (you have the experience by dint of the body you have) and embedded within your society, culture, and environment.

Modern healthcare tries to divide the person up into physical and mental, and then further compartmentalise into body parts, systems, or conditions. Think of all the hospital departments, and often separate buildings for the mind. It is convenient to deliver care and treatment this way and can work as long as the person comes first and communication between departments is smooth and up to date.

So, if you are suffering persistent pain (chronic pain or ongoing pain), this book has been written to help you understand your pain before looking at ways you can shape a positive future. The approach I take is person-first, coming through a compassionate lens within a framework that comes at understanding pain and health from a predictive and enactive perspective (Kiverstein et al., 2022; Miller et al., 2021; de Haan, 2020; Stilwell & Harman, 2019).

Of course, at the moment, these are just words. The following sections will make sense of the words and bring them alive in practical ways for you.

The people who come to see me or reach out from across the globe tell me about their unique experiences of pain and symptoms, for example:

- back pain
- neck pain
- complex regional pain syndrome (CRPS)

- irritable bowel syndrome (IBS)
- headaches
- migraines
- arthritis
- inflammatory conditions
- auto-immune conditions
- pelvic pain
- vulvodynia
- trigeminal neuralgia
- sports injuries (that have not got better as expected)
- post-surgery
- whiplash associated disorder (WAD)
- fibromyalgia
- chronic fatigue syndrome (CFS)
- myalgic encephalomyelitis (ME)
- neuropathic pain
- tendon pain
- anterior knee pain
- patellofemoral joint pain
- hip and groin pain
- chronic widespread pain
- Long COVID

There will be other reasons, and importantly, listening to people's narratives reveals a rich lived experience that the constructs listed above do not illustrate.

Some people have a number of seemingly different conditions or pains. However, there is always a commonality in that it is you, the person, who feels the pain and symptoms. There is also a common biology involving integrated body systems doing what they can to ensure you are healthy and surviving.

In other words, there is an overarching biological dynamic that underpins your experiences of pain in all the places that you feel it. This means we can address certain aspects of your biology, your thinking, and your lifestyle to go upstream to the source rather than just use a sticky plaster. Together we seek your transformation and growth, which is entirely possible, starting with understanding your pain and yourself.

This book is also for people who work with or care for people suffering persistent pain, so that they can understand what they can do to help. You could be a healthcare professional, an educator of professional helpers and carers, a case manager or have another role that brings you into contact with people who are suffering persistent pain.

--

I wanted to mention another term that is used: medically unexplained symptoms, or medically unexplained pain. This is used when the investigations and tests fail to show any pathology or injury that explains the pain. As you will see, the modern model for pain that I describe accounts for the fact that it is possible to have a negative test despite having pain. It is essential that we can account for your experience of pain and symptoms as well as any objective measure or scientific finding. The complete picture needs meaning and explanation.

One of the problems with the term is that if medicine is unable to explain your pain, then it is deemed to be psychological, psychosomatic, or something else. Unfortunately, even with the advances in understanding, you only need to read about people's experiences of appointments to realise that far too many remain unheard and dismissed in this way. This must change.

It is encouraging that more doctors are thinking about the person, lifestyle, and other important factors. We are moving away (slowly) from the idea that persistent pain is owned by medicine and that most of the practical work is done with therapists such as physiotherapists, occupational therapists, nurses, and psychologists who are trained to help. This is of course, once anything sinister has been eliminated, which medicine has a vital role in confirming.

Medicine offers a range of medications and interventions. These can be useful, and you may have gained some benefits. This type of treatment can be part of a programme of care, but it is only a part. Taking pain medication does not teach you how to move, live, look after yourself, or address the root causes. Going upstream is vital to gaining freedom. This takes understanding, self-awareness, self-care, self-compassion, and daily practical habits, the types that are detailed in the following section. None of these are selfish.

Typically, medicine uses a range of tests to establish a diagnosis. However, a reliance on these tests over and above the narrative shared by the person means that people suffering chronic pain, fibromyalgia, ME (myalgic encephalomyelitis), chronic fatigue syndrome (CFS), and Long COVID have endured disbelief and been told that it is psychological when tests show no disease state.

Further, people with CFS have been advised to use graded exercise because 'nothing is wrong with them', only to discover that the symptoms and suffering worsen. You only need to spend a short time with someone with ME/CFS to realise that there is an issue with their energy amongst other things, which will be underpinned by a biology that is yet to be fully understood.

Fortunately, there are continual advances in understanding the biology of pain and conditions such as ME/CFS. In particular, the role of the immune system has been confirmed (Tracey, 2021; Grace et al., 2014), issues with the energy-producing parts of cells identified (Morris & Maes, 2014), and the potential role of the gut microbiome (Konig et al., 2022), which offers explanations and treatment possibilities.

Now we have Long COVID, which is characterised by many similar symptoms (Aiyegbusi et al., 2021). Again, we are seeing people being dismissed because tests do not show anything of note. This is blatantly ignoring the person, failing to listen and validate their story. This highlights the nature of the problem: misunderstanding. But it is not just misunderstanding of Long COVID or chronic pain that is a major issue, it is also the fact that clinicians fall back on their own biases and limited beliefs. Again, this must change.

The person suffering is not to blame, although they may feel that way—I hope you don't. For clinicians, there is nothing wrong with not knowing the answers, but this must be admitted and the person be given some ideas about where to go next. This I think, would be preferable to the many negative messages given.

The way that you are treated, whether you feel heard and validated are all playing a role in the pain experience are shaping your expectations of future treatment. A further important consideration is the way that women, different ethnic groups, and the LGBTQ community are treated by healthcare. This is an enormous subject, which goes beyond the scope of this book. Gender bias is well documented (see Pain and Prejudice by Gabrielle Jackson, 2019) as are the issues with racial bias (Iacobucci, 2022; Meints et al., 2019; Hoffman et al., 2016; Meghani et al., 2012). This includes false beliefs about biological differences and undertreatment for pain.

When I listen to people's stories about their experiences and symptoms, despite seeing many people, often they don't know what is wrong. At the first meeting, no one has been able to fully explain their pain experience to me yet. Maybe that is you as well. We (the healthcare community) must make sense of your experiences and any tests that have been performed. This is the starting point—to validate and give meaning to your story by recognising you as a human being who is doing the best that you can with the knowledge and skills you have, grounded in your life view and past experiences. We must meet you where you are and start there rather than impose some model or framework upon you.

You are doing your best. I repeat.

If you want to understand your pain using the latest thinking in pain science and philosophy, and then look at ways of easing your suffering together with building health, this is for you.

How to use this book?

To help you, I have based this book on the sessions I have with people face to face and online. Whilst I am not actually in the room with you, I hope you get a sense of me being there with you on your journey. This is a collaboration.

My role is as a listener, a guide and an encourager. This is the essence of great coaching.

You might tell your story out loud now, imagining that I am there with you in the room, listening. If you do, how does that feel? To tell your story without being judged.

Once you have clarified your picture(s) of success, you can then choose the tools and practices that will take you in that direction.

There are three sections. The first will help you understand your pain and other experiences you may be having. The second guides you to be clear on what you want to achieve and why it matters. The third section describes skills, tools, exercises, and strategies that you can weave into your life as a practice, together with the know-how. They can sit alongside any existing useful practices and exercises you are using, that is, the ones that work for you. And together with other healthcare professionals.

It is not enough to just give someone some exercises to do and wish for the best. We need to know-how we implement the practices in our own world to get our best results.

Throughout the book there are 'Encouragement Points' at the end of each section, which are designed to keep you on track as you move on—encouraging you. They are not a full summary, but offer key insights.

The purpose of my work and this book is to help you to get better and improve your life by reconnecting with the important things: people, your sense of purpose, the planet, and your body.

As you create and curate your own programme, you may find it useful to keep a log of your successes. The wins you achieve each day are a key part of getting better. This is evidence that you can be successful and that there are times when you feel good and experience pleasure and joy. As humans, we often generalise how the day has been according to the peaks and troughs rather than an accurate picture of nuance and variability. Having insights into your actual experience is one of the important ways you can become unstuck. I have shared some practical aspects of using a log or journal below.

On purpose, this is a very practical book. I encourage you to be a full participant, using the suggested practices and implementation skills to immerse yourself in the experiences. This way you will gain the full richness of the results you create through your own endeavours.

The many skills and strategies described in the book are ways to create the conditions for a positive future; the one you desire. Of course, we must always be realistic, but positively so. This means that we focus on the things we want to achieve and take steps each day in that direction, in the best way that we can. One go at a skill is not the end result. It is a step.

I wish you well.

The journal

Your journal is a record of your wins and successes. This is the place for you to write down what has gone well that day. This is your evidence, helping you to see the bigger picture and actively switch to sampling the pleasures and joys that life offers, rather than just suffering.

This is not a pain diary for the simple reason that it gets you to focus on what you don't want rather than what you do want—pain. Writing down all the times when you are in pain means that this becomes the lens you look through.

Don't think of elephants.

Exactly.

One of the important life principles is that you should try to focus on what you want as much of the time as you can. You walk in the direction that the path takes, where you want to go, not into the wall at the side. In other words, you look where you are going, concentrating on this step right now.

One sunny afternoon I was running along a South Downs trail. It was very uneven, with lots of loose stones of varying sizes. The path started to course downwards steeply towards a gate. I wanted to get to the gate. At that moment, I realised a useful analogy. Yes, I wanted to arrive at the gate but I knew that to do so, rather than fall over (quite likely—I have had many a fall…), I needed to really focus on the step I was taking now and the next. By taking care of the moment and this step, I would most likely arrive where I wanted to. This is a good example of focusing on process over prize, an important principle for overcoming pain that has its own section.

I find that most people use their journal each day, jotting down two or three things they have done successfully. Some go beyond this and describe their actions in more detail. They also note why they think those things went well and what it felt like, bringing it alive with their words.

Even further, I have known people to draw, sketch, and write poems.

This is your journal, so you can use it however you like. But it is based on encouragement, giving you energy and empowering you to keep going in your chosen direction. When you return to read your entries, you should feel encouraged to keep going in your chosen direction. This is a route of mastery. Mastery of your life that has no ending in mind, instead a series of achievements and learning opportunities as you grow. If you look at anyone who has achieved success, they do not stop in their practice. They simply continue with what works well. You can do the same.

Digital journals are available on our devices. Yet there is something about a pen or pencil and a journal you can hold in your hands, carry in your pocket or bag.

At the front you state your pictures of success in clear terms, using positive language: focus on what you want. These you can read each day as a primer to your approach, giving you direction. Then you choose your intent and style.

After even a few weeks, the journal becomes a source of your successes to study. How can I continue to build on these wins and maintain momentum towards my picture(s) of success?

On the whole, you will be self-coaching as you are with you all the time. The journal is an excellent aid to help you keep focusing on what you can do, working towards your goals, having daily wins and a place where you can record inspiring quotes and ideas. It is a companion in your pocket that guides and prompts wise actions based on what is working for you.

Section 4 What is pain?

Contents

Understand pain

Pain is an enormous global issue affecting millions of people and costing billions. The suffering is immeasurable. You can think of it as a public health and social issue. This is a suffering society with increasing numbers of people enduring chronic illnesses emerging from a socioeconomic culture that puts profit over people, competition over cooperation, individualism over togetherness, and pleasure (quick fixes) over happiness (sustained). We are embedded in such an environment and its messages. Pain is experienced by the person within this environment where nature and values are ignored at the expense of trying to fit in and be accepted, which is a human need. Suffering is the cost.

It is estimated that 100 million Europeans (SIP, 2017), 100 million Americans, and 15.5 million people in England (Versus Arthritis, 2021) suffer from persistent pain. These are the people who are known about. The data analysis of the Health Survey for England on chronic pain by Public Health England and the charity versus arthritis looked at different age groups and found the most worrying trend in 16–34-year-olds. The proportion of people suffering chronic pain in that age group has risen from 21% to 34%. A more recent paper charted a worrying trend, showing an increase in the percentage of people in pain across 146 countries, from 26.3% in 2009 to 32.1% in 2021 (Macchia, 2022).

Whilst technology and the way we live are evolving at a rapid rate, so is suffering. This is in part, perhaps a large part, down to the way we think about pain in our society. And perhaps a loss of meaning. A listlessness for a range of reasons beyond the scope of exploration here but nonetheless important.

Most of the care is based on the biomedical model, which does not explain pain experiences. We have known this since the 1960s when Professor Pat Wall and Ron Melzack came up with the Gate Theory of Pain (Melzack & Wall, 1965). Since this time, scientists and people who study pain have stood on shoulders and more shoulders to bring us to what we now think and understand about pain. This is ongoing work and we will discover more. Unfortunately, the pinnacle of this understanding is well in advance of what is practiced day to day in society and healthcare. This gap needs to be closed and is one of the major challenges we face.

In a seminal paper 'On the relation of injury and pain' by Wall in 1979, he stated:

> *Pain is better classified as an awareness of a need-state than as a sensation. It serves more to promote healing than to avoid injury. It has more in common with the phenomena of hunger and thirst than it has with seeing or hearing. The period after injury is divided into the immediate, acute and chronic stages. In each stage it is shown that pain has only a weak connection to injury but a strong connection to the body state.*

> *'I often say to people, pain is less reflective of the area that hurts and more reflective of how you are in your current situation (literally this minute).' RS*

That was over 40 years ago, but still society predominantly considers pain and injury to be well-related, even interchangeably using the terms at times. Not only is this wrong, but it takes people down the wrong path in terms of what they do and expect.

The biomedical approach searches for structural, pathological, or other measurable and visible causes for pain. For example, the belief that seeing a disc injury on a scan can be deemed the source of pain. But there is a fundamental issue with this thinking—you cannot see pain. Pain is subjective and can only ever be experienced by the person uniquely and privately. There is no test that shows pain. Much like there is no test that shows hunger. They are felt experiences and purely subjective. Only you can feel your pain. The idea that 'I can feel your pain' is simply untrue.

Despite these insights, the biomedical model predominates. It seems to make sense according to our experiences, and we have been conditioned and encultured to believe it. This can even be the case in the face of hard data. A recent study with 3369 participants showed MRI findings in people with and without back pain. A longitudinal analysis found that most of these findings were not associated with low back pain in the future (Kasch et al., 2022). Contrast this to many people's beliefs that their persistent pain will continue. This is the story that they become locked into through their own beliefs and expectations, which have been shaped by society's messages and things they have been told by health-care professionals.

The power of beliefs and expectations is immense. They are shaped for each of us uniquely as we go through life, delivered by caregivers (including parents, family), educators, social media, and society. This is why they must be accurate, based on the facts and not opinions, together with insights into the nature of being and life. For example, inter-being and impermanence (Thich Nhat Hanh, 2017) that we will look at later. There are two layers: understanding the pain as a unique experience and the context. The latter includes your life so far and life's realities. Both need to be considered to gain the best picture of where the onward journey begins.

A model to explain pain must be able to account for all scenarios including clear scans, investigations that do not reveal anything noteworthy (despite there being pain and other symptoms), phantom limb pain, and congenital insensitivity to pain (CIP) (Goldberg, 2007). CIP is a rare genetic condition when the person does not experience pain. Further, it must give meaning to the variability of experiences between people and the different experiences the person is having. How painful can a paper cut be? Why do some people not feel pain when they have suffered serious injury? Why does a movement hurt one day and less so or more the next? Why does it hurt when the scan reveals nothing?

These are the questions that must be answered. The biomedical model cannot do this, so the person and the clinicians who subscribe to this thinking continue their search with more tests and investigations. Meanwhile, the worry and concern build as expectations and hopes continue to be dashed. This in itself is a factor for developing persistent pain as I will explain, together with the feelings of not being heard or believed.

Of course, it is important to rule out serious pathology or a disease that needs specific treatment. There will be certain tests that may need to be performed but must be done together with listening to and validating your narrative and experience. Once this has been done, the focus can turn to easing suffering and creating a practice to build wellness and live your best life.

Pain in 2023—drawing from multiple fields

'Pain is what and where you say it is'

~ my take on the classic definition by Margo McCaffery of 1968

You may have heard of the biopsychosocial (BPS) model (Engel, 1977; 1980). This was an attempt to widen thinking about the person to consider their biology, psychology, and social circumstances. Undoubtedly, this offers more than the biomedical model that does not see or acknowledge the whole person, their experiences, and circumstances—the complexity of health conditions is not addressed.

I would like to emphasise here that the issue is with the model itself and the system in which it continues to be used and not the clinicians. Many therapists, doctors, and allied health professionals have a human and caring approach, even coming through the biomedical lens. They genuinely want to help and become frustrated when their offerings have little or no impact. There are inherent biases in the system that need realising and weeding out.

Whilst the BPS model appears to cover the bases, it has limitations (Stilwell & Harman, 2019). There is a tendency for clinicians to revert to the 'bio' (the biology) to explain pain. Further, there can be a false separation between the dimensions in its application rather than exploring where they meet as your lived experience. Essentially, what we need is a way of incorporating the objective and the subjective. Or put another way, an approach that brings together your subjective experience of pain and what can be seen and tested scientifically. This has always been the challenge, and now it appears that we have such an approach as you will see in the coming sections.

Bringing different disciplines together is often fruitful for complex issues. Pain is no exception. It is a great example of a perception or a conscious experience. Another is love, which you also cannot see. Or hunger. But few doubt the experience. Arguably then, we must understand how and why we perceive, and how it comes to be that we are conscious, to understand pain. There has been renewed interest in consciousness science and a thirst for comprehending the human condition at a deeper level, perhaps because it seems that society is suffering more. Scientists, philosophers, and writers such as Anil Seth, Andy Clark, Mick Thacker, and Mark Miller are leading the way in deepening our understanding, to name but a few.

In Western culture, suffering is viewed as something bad, whereas in Eastern culture, suffering is deemed a part of everyday life. I ask, who will suffer more as a consequence of their beliefs? I am unsurprised by the growing interest in Buddhism. Increasing comfort (housing, clothing, food, convenience) for many, not all, means that being comfortable with being uncomfortable has become a thing. Undoubtedly, the many advances in healthcare are benefiting society, but not when it comes to pain. Persistent or on-going pain continues to be a huge problem (Goldberg & McGee, 2011). Part of this is due to the way we think about pain. I hasten to add that this is not about blaming individuals, a culture, or society, instead understanding all the contributing factors to the enormous levels of suffering so that we can do better.

In terms of pain, it has become a human right to be given pain relief. This is a massive challenge because, despite years of trying, medicine has been unable to deliver consistent and acceptable results. Tie this with each person's individual take on their own situation, and the complexity emerges. Some people's expectations are more in line with their realities, allowing them to move forward. This is desirable to make positive changes along with flexibility and openness to possibility.

Other people have expectations of themselves that are too high, considering their circumstances, resulting in repeated failures to succeed. This seems to be a contributing factor to the stuckness with pain. Neither is this the person's fault, as all of our expectations are conditioned—we did not and are not choosing to think that way. But on realisation, it is our responsibility to do the best we can. Having said that, there are other variables such as access to care and whether that care is in line with the latest thinking in pain. Essentially, you are always doing the best with the skills that you have, but you may need more. Whether you can get that help or not is a social concern.

We need different thinkers to get together. Fortunately, this is happening with philosophy and science as I mentioned. You might be wondering about the existing multidisciplinary teams (MDT) thinking that they provide an example of different healthcare professionals working together. That is true, they do. But despite these teams, there is still a growing pain problem and predicted to worsen (Ferreira et al., 2023, Macchia, 2022).

Partly, there are not enough dedicated services with true pain specialists in the field (people with specific training in pain science and treatment with the necessary skill set), and partly it will be the way that they work. For example, it has not been uncommon for pain management courses run by MDTs that start by saying that they are not there to help with the pain. Instead, the focus is on coping. To me, this is demotivating and wrong. We should be helping the person get better and improve their life, including easing pain, suffering, and symptoms. Coping with difficult moments is important, but not the main thrust.

So what do I mean by other disciplines? The best working example, because it has been happening and delivering new thinking with practical applications, is the collaboration between scientists, philosophers, and clinicians.

The philosophers bring new and better questions and thinking for the scientists to prove or disprove. This togetherness and collaboration was just what was needed for pain, and now we have ways of thinking that can offer great hope. The ongoing work and studies of one of my greatest influences, Professor Mick Thacker in particular, together with Julian Kiverstein, Karl Friston, Andy Clark, Mark Miller, Peter Stilwell, Inês Hipólito, Anna Ciaunica, and Sabrina Coninx are especially notable. There are others of course. Together they are shaping a contemporary way of thinking about pain grounded in a long history of philosophy and neuroscience.

Previously a range of other models were put forward to explain pain. These included the Mature Organism Model (Gifford, 1998), the Fear Avoidance Model (Vlaeyen & Linton, 2000), the pain neuromatrix (Melzack, 2001), and the Salience Detection System for the body (Legrain et al., 2011). All these contributions were important to develop our understanding, which is an ongoing journey.

The advent of functional MRI scanning meant that researchers and scientists could look at brain activity when people were experiencing pain. From this, they could assume that certain brain cell patterns were a representation of pain. In other words, a neural substrate of what people were feeling. This put the brain at the forefront of pain research, clarifying the so-called pain matrix. The pain matrix is the term used to describe a network of areas of the brain that would be active if the person was in pain.

This fascinating and revealing research featuring brain regions in different colours was compelling (e.g. Tracey & Martyr, 2007; Baliki et al., 2012; Mansour et al., 2014). It led to and developed ideas about focusing on and retraining the brain, tied with the understanding of neuroplasticity, the brain's ability to change. In 1949, the Canadian psychologist Donald Hebb was reported to have said for the first time that neurons that fire together, wire together. He was referring to neurons that repeatedly communicate and forge increasingly effective signalling—they work better. The plastic ability of the nervous system meant that we could learn, increasing our abilities with repetition, or practice.

Brain-based research continues to evolve with the refinement of techniques and the quality of the equipment. Whilst this is contributing to the field, it is by no means the only consideration. We must be able to put this into the perspective of our experience, otherwise it is meaningless, and goes beyond the brain—we are more than a brain.

A further issue that has been highlighted is the quality of the studies. Recent work has pointed out the problem with the number of subjects in fMRI studies

(Grady et al., 2020). Looking at this, the authors concluded that 'the sample size commonly used in fMRI studies of 20–30 participants is very unlikely to be sufficient for obtaining reproducible brain-behaviour correlations, regardless of analytic approach'. From this, we are compelled to carefully consider study findings and conclusions, particularly those of prior studies that have influenced treatment approaches or the understanding of pain.

Many clinicians and therapists were excited by ideas of brain changes because they appeared to give an explanation for what they were doing and seeing. They could tell their patients that the exercises and treatments work by changing their brain. And by changing their brain, they could change their pain. This is still a popular message. It is entirely understandable and makes sense.

There are now many apps that offer brain training explanations for their existence, much like those that offer such training to boost intelligence. Inevitably there will be people who claim that their pain has improved because of the app, but how do you really know? Of course, you don't. It is an opinion or a guess that the reason you feel better is because of the app rather than innumerable other variables. However, if you feel better, you feel better. What you tell yourself can become your reality through your own expectations bearing out. In other words, your expectations about getting better by using a particular programme are playing a role that could be greater than the app itself. We now have a wealth of evidence about the expectation effect, which we can skilfully harness (Robson, 2022). Brain training can appear to make sense. It seems logical. But there are a few issues with this thinking.

Your brain is undoubtedly an important organ. But there is more to you and much more to pain than the brain. For instance, in Karl Friston's words, the brain is embodied, it lives in a body, it uses a body (Embodied Cognition: Serious Science, 2019). There is not much we can do without a body! Wherever you find yourself, whatever you are doing, there is your body, playing a big role in how you feel, think, perceive, and act. Put another way, you think, act, and perceive the world in your own way because of the particular body that you have. The opportunities or affordances that appear to you do so because you have a body. But as with the brain, you are more than a body. And you exist in an environment. So, you are better to think of the 'body-brain-environment' to get closer to reality. Going beyond the brain and neurons to consider the whole person is an important move, which better explains what is seen and felt. Body systems work in a far more complex and dynamic way that the textbooks would suggest.

For example, the nervous, endocrine, and immune systems are more accurately thought of as an ensemble, like a music band, and appear to be playing a role in your thinking as part of how your biology self-organises in a particular situation, behaving and adopting in a way that supports ongoing goals being achieved and of course survival (Ciaunica et al., 2023; Clark, 2023).

Both our experiences and science now agree that the brain and body are entwined, as opposed to being separate (dualism or Cartesian) with the sense of our bodies giving us information about how we are (Clark, 2023; Tsakiris & De Preester, 2019). In fact, we can go further and embrace embodied cognition, which is 'the idea that the mind is not only connected to the body but that the body influences the mind' (McNerney, 2011).

With the knowledge that we have now, the surprising element is that generally, medicine and healthcare continue to separate mind, body, and brain. This highlights the challenge of updating beliefs and ways of thinking. Essentially, we are seeking to replace a simple idea with a more complex one, something that Pat Wall, the father of modern pain science and medicine, acknowledged as a significant challenge many years ago. And here we are continuing to try to help society move forward with its thinking about pain. To do that, we need people to understand their own experiences as unified.

In other words, the body, mind, brain, and environment are not interrelated or even connected. Together they form the experience. This becomes apparent when you look more closely, such as when meditating. Otherwise, they appear to be separate because that is the belief in Western culture. Beliefs shape how things appear.

This matters because separating them out misses the opportunities to see things as they are and to take skilful action. Knowing that what you are doing, what you are perceiving and thinking all come together because of each other gives you a huge range of options as you will see. Underpinning this is biology of course, some of which is now understood.

For example, there is good evidence that inflammation underpins depression and the sickness response (Dantzer et al., 2008), which has been known for some years. The immune system is responsible for inflammatory processes, but very much works together with the nervous and endocrine systems. This ties in with chronic stress that essentially results in chronic inflammation as the body switches into an ongoing healing mode because there is a perceived threat to integrity. Biologically this makes sense, although often there is no actual threat. It is imagined via a thought, which is often automatic. You are not choosing to think about certain things, they just pop in with an accompanying feeling state.

Think of a time when you felt anxious. Was the thing you were anxious about actually happening? If you are engaged with the thought of that unpleasant or scary future, your body prepares for it, mobilising resources that you feel as bodily sensations. Then you interpret those sensations: I'm anxious. That is what it becomes. And it does so through repetition or habit of thought based on your underlying beliefs about yourself and the world. So, it goes a bit deeper than you may think. But within this is an opportunity to understand, let go, and be free of suffering.

The effects of chronic stress are well understood (Sapolsky, 2004). Every body's system is affected. The sickness response mentioned above is inflammation in action. You will be familiar with this from having the flu, but it is also a common feature of chronic pain, whiplash-associated disorder, fibromyalgia, ME, and CFS. People have been describing these feelings but do not seem to be given the explanation as to why. Now we can. The body is responding as if sick, with the same chemicals and the same feelings. There are many studies showing the involvement of the immune system and inflammation in painful and psychiatric conditions (e.g. Alshelh et al., 2022; Beurel et al., 2020; Daniels et al., 2020; Bauer & Teixeira, 2019).

This being the case, we can think about ways to address inflammation in the person's life. For example, by reconnecting with what matters (people, purpose, the planet), learn better ways to manage stress and anxiety (skills), prioritising self-care, and perhaps anti-inflammatory medication (Malys & Mondelli, 2022).

With your immune system and other body systems continually anticipating, predicting, and acting to maintain your biology within narrow parameters, the awareness of this is the felt sense: How am I right now? The way you feel emerges from the way your systems are sensing the environment in which you find yourself (what is happening now), prior experiences in that environment, your beliefs, emotions, and expectations, all coming together, making sense of what is happening for you. Much of this is subconscious processing, so you don't need to be thinking certain thoughts, although you might be: 'Will that chair be comfortable?' You just have the conscious experience that appears without effort.

So, this is complex. Much more than the biomedical model might assume. But through this complexity and understanding your experiences more fully, you will begin to see the opportunities to transform suffering using the practices and strategies in the book.

All of what I have been explaining is happening in your body and by the fact that you have the body that you do, in this moment—experiences are embodied. I am hoping that you can start to see how 'the whole' comes together and why we must draw upon different fields to understand and then take positive action.

Embodiment is your actual experience. You have a body that enables you to act upon and experience the world. It is predicted, expected, and known— 'this is me'. Your body contributes hugely to the sense of who you are; your 'self' if you like. You might like to take a moment to pause and notice what it is like to be you right now. What are your reference points? This can feel a little strange if you are not used to this kind of practice. In meditation, it is common to experience the loss of sense of self. It somehow dissolves, which may sound scary!

Being present and aware is the realm of contemplation (e.g. meditation, mindfulness, prayer). This may be something you practice. It has become very popular in the West, but often for the wrong reasons. Mindfulness, for example, is a way of being: open, aware, present, non-judgemental. It is not something you do to get somewhere or be someone special. Being mindful means that you have insights into the nature of being and reality. You see and experience things how they are rather than through the distortions of your embodied mind. This kind of practice creates the conditions for freedom from suffering. But if you practice in order to become free, you are not present. See the paradox?

There is immense value in such practices as part of our lives. They can easily be integrated into the day to day. To back this as a healthy way of being, there has been a great deal of research in recent years. Some of this has been driven by the openness and curiosity of Buddhist leaders such as the Dalai Lama and Thich Nhat Hahn who have encouraged scientific study.

Scientists have also been interested to discover more, in particular Francisco Varela and Evan Thompson, who proposed a new way of studying the neuro-science of consciousness (2001). They described their approach that 'allows for theories and hypotheses about the two-way or reciprocal relationship between embodied conscious states and local neuronal activity'. This chimes well with the need to account for scientific findings and your experience of pain and other symptoms.

Many other scientists and philosophers are seeking to understand percep-tion, cognition, and action as a lived experience from different perspectives (e.g. Noë, 2004; Dum et al., 2019). Our role as scientific clinicians is to critically appraise the work and distil it into something practical and use-ful to ease your suffering. One area of study that has gained momentum is interoception, which is the sense of your internal physiology (Garfinkel et al., 2014).

We understand the importance of the embodied feeling of existence that is typically taken for granted. Why would you think about it? Until it changes or disappears. Or you become over-focused on certain sensations. Most people will have such an experience and in some it persists. This is called depersonalisation and derealisation when things feel unreal and you feel detached from your body and the world (Ciaunica & Charlton, 2018).

These experiences can be most peculiar and in some cases alarming when you don't know what is happening. In fact, together with illusions, they demonstrate the fragility of our experiences, supporting the notion that we are actively constructing our perceptions rather than being a passive recipient (Seth, 2021). When I am listening to a person telling me their story, I want to know about them, as they are impacting their quality of life. This is what we are seeking to change. Hence feeling more whole, more present, more aware are all signs of being better and healthier.

Knee pain. Where does it hurt? In your brain or your knee? Some people have been told that it is in their brain. When I ask 'Where in their brain?', they are stumped. Pain involves the brain, but it is not and cannot be 'in' the brain. Others take this message as meaning pain is in their head and therefore not real. This can have a detrimental effect when we know the importance of being seen, heard and your story being validated.

Believing that your pain is in your brain has another effect. If it is in there somehow, how can I do something about it? Again, this is reducing the experience to one organ or a pattern of activity, despite the fact that the actual lived experience is embodied—you feel it in your body. There is nothing about your head that is felt in relation to knee pain. If you examine your own experience, you come to know this as true.

The explanations that we give to you about your pain must make sense and relate to your actual experience of what it is like to be in pain. Reducing pain in the brain is no better in that way than reducing it to a ligament or muscle, colourful illustrations of brain activity, or a list of statistics. We can account for all of these objective findings, but only within the bigger picture of the person's descriptions of the subjective nature of their pain, within a particular context and environment. Anything less is an incomplete explanation with consequences: ongoing confusion, misunderstanding, concerns and worries, and less-than-optimal choices.

Understand pain: Why?

'Understanding your pain is the first step to overcoming pain. Understanding changes your beliefs, which changes your pain experience.' RS

You may have a good idea why understanding your pain is important from your own experiences as well as what I have said. You want, need, and deserve an explanation that fits what it is like for you. It must make sense and resonate with you so that you can see a way forward and feel hope.

In my opinion, understanding your pain and other symptoms is the first step. Spending time talking about your experiences and having them explained in plain language sets the scene for the things you can do to move forward.

The beliefs that you have about your pain have built up from a very early stage in life. Bumps, bruises, and injuries along the way from childhood, together with the way caregivers responded and the types of messages they gave you, will have shaped your beliefs. These in turn play a role in your actual perception of pain; what it is like for you. This can be difficult to take on board when we have often been brought up to think that pain is well-related to injury or damage, and because of the way it actually feels.

Knowing that thoughts, past experiences, expectations, the current situation you find yourself in, emotions and mood merge to create your lived world helps in my view. Of course, we have no access to the way in which our systems do this, just the raw experience itself. Or as philosopher, cognitive scientist and happiness aficionado Dr. Mark Miller puts it in his TEDx talk, we just have the crunch when it all comes together. This is your perception. But your reality is your perception.

Many people I meet have moved on from the pain equals injury kind of thinking, but are still stuck with their pain. I often ask people to think about it: What do you really think is happening? This is because we can take on board a new perspective, but it remains superficial. Deep down, you are not yet convinced or a part of you keeps questioning it. This can be part of the stuckness, and you need some practical experience to update your beliefs and thinking.

You may be stuck with both persistent pain and a belief that there must be an injury or pathology. Tests may have been negative so far, or shown little to explain your symptoms, yet you continue to seek something physical to explain them. A test result, a definite diagnosis, or something to show is needed to make it real in your mind.

In recent years, work and research have shown the variance in tissue state and pain, highlighting other important factors and predictors for persistent pain. Osteoarthritis (OA) is typically thought of as wear and tear of the joints (cartilage), causing inflammation, pain, and stiffness. Now we know that it is far more complex involving the subchondral bone and the synovium (the lining of the joint), which release inflammatory molecules together with metabolic syndrome and immune system contributions to sensitivity (Berenbaum, 2013). OA is not just about the painful joint. It is a whole-person issue relating to past experiences, lifestyle, context, expectations, beliefs, and other health factors.

A cohort of people with rheumatoid arthritis, an autoimmune condition, was studied to determine the trajectories of their pain predicted by certain baseline characteristics (McWilliams et al., 2019). The authors concluded that there were subgroups of people who each had a different pain prognosis. Interestingly, the risk factors for persistent pain were a smoking history and high disability. They also discovered that pain was ongoing when inflammation resolved. In other words, inflammation is not the only factor to consider.

Back pain is a very common problem causing much distress and suffering. Often parts of the spine are blamed for the pain: for example, facet joints, discs. Many people have scans to look for a cause of their pain, which of course you cannot see (you can't see pain). Yet the association between degenerative findings on a scan and back pain is hugely varied. For instance, we know that some people can have disc injuries but no pain. A recent study of over 3000 people concluded that MRI degenerative findings 'did not have clinically important associations with low back pain' (Kasch et al., 2022).

The evidence for other factors is far stronger. For instance, one study that looked at the structural and psychosocial factors for low back pain (100 participants who had mild persistent low back pain) over a 4–6 year period (Carragee et al., 2005). The authors found that the psychosocial variables were far more predictive of serious disability than the state of the body tissues (structures). This is unsurprising when you consider the fact that we do not have a direct experience of our bodies or the world. Instead, we perceive ourselves and the world as a best guess (Seth, 2022). There are many variables that feed into this perception including past experiences, beliefs, context, and expectations.

Tendon pain and injury have been well studied over the years, largely focusing on the tendon itself down to a microscopic level. Despite this work, many people continue to struggle with tendon problems. Similar to other persistent pains, the solution is to zoom out, not in. Understanding the person and the context is vital. A recent piece of research looked at people with gluteal tendinopathy, the most common of the lower limbs, to establish which factors are important (Plinsinga et al., 2018). Interestingly, there was no difference in local muscle strength between those with severe and mild symptoms. However, they did find that those with more severe pain experienced higher levels of catastrophising and depression, and lower self-efficacy and quality of life.

Whilst the strength of the relationship is uncertain, and as ever we need more high-quality studies, I would argue that the person and their circumstances must be considered with any pain problem. These are the basis for the existence of pain in the first place and provide the context, past experiences, beliefs, and expectations that emerge as perceptions of self and the world. At the end of the day, this is what we are seeking to sustainably change for the better, shaping a positive future.

Plenty of other studies support these findings, which means that we have to go beyond the tissues to understand pain. You simply cannot understand a person or their lived experience from seeing a disc, a ligament, or a muscle. This is not to say that the tissues are not important; they are! They need to be healthy with a good blood and oxygen supply and plenty of movement. But there is a difference between the tissues and the experience of oneself in the world. And whilst this is more complex, it offers many opportunities to overcome pain.

The question of being believed often comes up in conversation. Without something to show others, how do you prove that you feel pain? If you are wearing a sling, have a wound, or even a limp, there is something demonstrable. But you may not have anything to point to in order to convince others of your pain.

I always wonder why you should have to prove it beyond what you say? When you speak of hunger or tiredness, there is no question about whether you are actually feeling it or not. So why is there ever doubt with pain?

Many people who I see feel that they have not been heard. You may relate to this in your own experience. Your symptoms, description of what it is like for you, and the impact on your life may have been dismissed in favour of objective tests and measures that show little. This can be confusing and certainly upsetting when you want to know why you continue to feel pain and suffer, and to know what you can do. In fact, when you are not taken seriously, this adds to your suffering and can diminish hope for a better future.

A diagnosed condition can add a perceived credibility or perhaps realness in your eyes that does not exist in the same way as something more vague. There appears to be a definite pathology and often a treatment or a path to follow. You can give the name of the condition to someone and explain what you are doing about it. This seems simple and is easily accepted. Without such a diagnosis, what do you say? Persistent or chronic pain is a label, but do people know what it means to you? It can be very difficult to explain, even to loved ones. This is the reason I have included a section on this (Family and Friends).

This particular issue highlights the importance of understanding pain. When you understand pain, you know that there is never anything to be seen. You know that although there is nothing visible, it is always real. It has been called an invisible illness. I am not sure about this description. To say it is invisible may again be suggestive that it is not real, but to you it is your reality.

In summary, understanding your pain helps you to give meaning to your experiences, to be able to explain to others what you are dealing with and how, and to engage with the many ways that you can shape a positive future. You have the insight that your experiences are your particular version of circumstances, that you have a body in the world, yet your perception of those is not a direct representation. Just a best guess, which is good enough.

Now I will discuss the position we can take on pain (2023), outlining the framework that we can use to understand pain and hence the sorts of practices, tools, and exercises you can use.

Embodied Predictive Processing (EPP)

Embodied predictive processing (EPP) is a contemporary model and way of thinking that can help us understand the lived experience of pain, put forward by the philosophers Julian Kiverstein and Michael Kirchhoff, and Mick Thacker, a neuroscientist with a background in physiotherapy (Kiverstein et al., 2021). It builds on predictive processing (PP) as a way of understanding being human in terms of action, perception, emotion, language, and learning (Nave et al., 2020), by recognising that there is more than the brain at play.

The excellent work by these authors is informing ways of thinking about pain that I believe are giving great hope. EPP gives us a way of explaining your experience and the scientific processes, including the neurobiology of pain, test results, and objective measures. In other words, we can account for the whole person and the whole picture in a way that other models cannot (the biomedical model, the biopsychosocial model).

We have a brain that is part of a body in a world, in a particular situation and environment where multiple opportunities exist for you, an individual. When pain is in the picture, these opportunities can diminish as can the sense of having choices without painful implications. In persistent pain, this becomes the lens through which life is seen and expected.

EPP has emerged from philosophy and science getting together. Philosophy knows how to ask questions and science knows how to investigate questions. They need each other. This is being borne out in academic papers, but more importantly, in practical ways that allow us to make sense of the person's lived experience and what is seen on tests and examinations. Bringing the subjective and the objective together is vital, building a complete picture before deciding upon a route forward.

Pain, like all perceptions, can be thought of as a prediction or an inference about what best explains the sense data and current situation for the person, based on prior experiences (see TED talk with Anil Seth and TEDx talk with Mick Thacker). When the prediction and the sense data match, there is nothing more that needs to be done. A perception is generated and we see the world as we expect to see it, including ourselves. There are no surprises.

However, when the prediction does not match the sense data, this creates a prediction error. Next, we seek to either change our model of the world by learning something new (perceptual inference), or act in such a way to gather new sense data that may then match the prediction (active inference)—we try to make better predictions. It is deemed adaptive and therefore good to be able to minimise these prediction errors over time, although the way we do this may not always be healthy as such.

There is a further important element: weighting or a weighing up. This means that your systems weigh towards the most reliable explanation for the current lived world. So, if you have experienced pain in a particular situation and there is something like that happening now, the past experience can be deemed a more reliable explanation, and hence this is your actual experience. The expectation is now that this context is painful (because it has been before), even if the sense data of that moment reports as within the normal parameters. Remember that what you perceive is your reality (it is real; it is happening), but it is a version of events unique to you, being generated top down.

An important example and point is that of feeling pain in the body (where else can you feel it?) in a location, that seems like it is coming from the body tissues, say your back. This is how it appears, just as it seems like the world is there in front of you. However, we now know that these experiences, in fact all experiences, are being generated top down. You will hear me talk about the map and the territory. We experience the map, not the territory, and at times we must update the map, otherwise we get lost. Many people I speak to who are suffering from chronic pain tell me they feel lost and want to find a path.

It is common to seek quick fixes to deal with pain, or in PP terms, to reduce the error. We are in a society with plenty of quick-fix offerings, which means they become expected for health as well. The problem is that there are no such solutions for persistent pain. So, you are in pain and find a way to ease it quickly, which in the short-term feels good, but is not in line with long-term healthy and valued goals. In fact, some quick fixes are harmful.

I use the example of alcohol below, but this could include medication use, especially opioids (e.g. morphine-based drugs). The error that is pain is rapidly reduced by using opiate medication, which is experienced as a significant relief. Great, you may think. Something that works for me! This is entirely understandable. However, although you are successfully minimising error, in the long-term, opiates can become addictive with all the associated problems. Skilful use of opiates for acute pain, on the other hand, managed and monitored closely, can be helpful.

Some people relieve their pain using alcohol. They feel better when they have a drink, and it becomes a strategy to minimise error, which feels good. Naturally, this can be a strategy used over and over to ease pain, but is in fact having other effects on the brain, body, and body systems that are not in line with being healthy and well. An important point around the use of alcohol or drugs is to know that there is and should not be any blame attached. The person, perhaps you, is doing their best with the resources that they have currently.

The key, then, is to find ways of minimising error with actions (exercises, movements, activities practices) that bring results and in the long term achieve wellness. In some cases, we can actually create an error on purpose that we seek to minimise. You might think of this as setting yourself a challenge or a goal that seems to be achievable. For example, going for a walk, choosing a distance or time that is within your window of tolerance, or a task at home. This is a route of mastery.

You will read about how you set yourself up for wins and successes in the practical sections of the book. This is an essential part of getting better, by creating the evidence that you can be successful and actually feel better. But you are doing this through your own experiments or tasks as well as being consciously aware of day-to-day successes.

How can you think about your pain?

How does this predictive model explain your pain that appears to have got stuck? The stickiness in part comes from repeatedly doing worse than expected. Initially you believe that you will get better, but then you don't. Treatments and exercises don't work despite your efforts. At some point, there is a switch from expecting to get better to expecting pain in different situations. Recall that we experience the world that we expect to experience.

Essentially, your systems are now looking out for evidence that you are in pain as opposed to evidence for getting better or being well. How do you know? Check out the thoughts and stories that you are listening to. What kind of picture are they painting for you? What is your outlook? Are you taking those thoughts as fact and the only possibility? How much do you pay attention to limiting beliefs? Again, if you are engaging with thoughts and stories about not getting better, it is not your fault. This is conditioning at play.

Now you can start applying the brakes. That story, that thought, how true is it? Are there other possibilities? The short answer is yes. The thoughts and stories are just that, thoughts and stories. No one actually knows the future, yet if you convince yourself of a particular (bleak) future, then you will seek the evidence to confirm it. That's the way you work as a human. But you can also have the insight about how this is working, then transcend and transform your suffering.

In this kind of stuckness, the world is now one full of possible and actual threats to your integrity, that is, damage. To your body systems, this now makes sense because of your prior experiences and is a much more reliable explanation than anything else that is going on for you. This can even be when there is no damage or risk of damage.

It is quite possible that you are in a 'no threat' state, which is being signalled via the complex network of systems and pathways in the body. But because past experiences have frequently been notable and impacting in terms of pain, this seems like a much more plausible explanation for what is happening now. The sense data that is saying 'we are ok' is ignored as noisy and unreliable. The result is pain, despite there being no actual danger or information suggesting a state of balance and wellness.

You will now recognise what I am describing here—the weighing-up process. Which seems more likely? Past experience or the current context? The types of things that push the weighting one way or another are expectations, attention, and prior notable events. Most people come to realise that the more they expect something to hurt, the more likely it will and often more intensely. Research backs up this experience that people describe (Jepma et al., 2018). An expectation is a thought but also occurs subconsciously within the processing of sensory information. So sometimes you may not be overtly thinking that it will hurt, but it does because your systems have predicted pain based on prior experiences in that type of situation, whilst largely ignoring other evidence. Pain makes the best sense of what is happening for you right now. Uncovering why this is the case is an important discovery, revealing your work.

Another way that you can push the weighting towards pain is by putting your attention on it. Thoughts and feelings about the pain in that moment will also flavour your experience. In a sense, there is a story that you tell yourself, which gives your pain a perspective, your unique perspective. But this is one of many possibilities, despite how convincing the story appears. You may have noticed how entangled you become with these thoughts until you have the insight that you are not the thoughts. You are the one who hears the thoughts. This creates some space for you to become disentangled and practice more skilful responses. These can be increasingly grounded in self-care and compassion as you transform your suffering.

We can work with both of these as part of the skill set to overcome pain as you will see.

This insight helps us understand the many times when you feel pain without there being any objective evidence for injury, pathology, or anything else that could be considered dangerous. But it also accounts for biology such as inflammation that can play a role in persistent pain states.

For instance, neurogenic inflammation occurs without injury, instead being a feature of sensitisation. In this case, your body (neuro-immune-endocrine ensemble) produces inflammatory molecules that are released in the tissues that are supplied by the involved neural pathways. The result can be the same as that of injury, the cardinal signs of heat, pain, swelling, and redness (you don't have to have all of these visibly).

This is when you notice that you are in pain having not done anything different or new and certainly not having injured yourself. As you know though, you can also experience pain without this happening if pain is deemed to be the best explanation for your lived world at that moment.

As I write this, I know that the complexity that I am bringing to you can sound very different from what you have previously been told and learned about pain. In one way I hope that this is the case because if you are reading this book, you have most likely not had much success with that approach. What I can say is that through this complexity arises many opportunities to move onwards.

So, you can think of your persistent pain as this kind of stuckness or a habitual perception that emerges from the ensemble of body systems to best explain what is happening for you in your lived world. Now you need another set of predictions and perceptions, which you have an active role in creating. This is the good news that brings much hope. The idea that you are somehow a passive recipient of the pain experience has been disproved. By the fact that you have a body and brain, you are enacting your pain in the way you think and move in particular situations and environments. And because you can think and move in many different ways, you can change your pain in many different ways. The understanding of how we enact our thoughts and feeling states with our bodies (Varela et al., 2017; Noë, 2004) has been revealing and offers a range of ways to generate new experiences with new thinking and actions

You can and are now deepening your understanding of your pain, which immediately starts to update your model and experience and take action to work towards your picture of success. You are actively creating that evidence by generating your perceptions (all of them including pain) with new knowledge and experiences. This creates possibilities as you realise your potential. You are not just a passenger on this life journey. Instead, you are the architect.

Considering pain as a perception that is being generated (see TED talk: Mick Thacker), like all of our experiences, helps you to position it as something you can influence, something you can ease, transform, and overcome. It may seem out of reach or impossible to you based on your experiences. This is why understanding pain in its most modern sense is so important because then it will begin to make sense to you. And you realise what you can do, think, and how you can act to move forward.

The reality is that the future, your future, is a blank slate. There are few absolute knowns. It is this uncertainty that makes life possible yet it creates such concern for people who have a need for certainty. With the future never coming, as there is only ever this moment, we have a choice as to how we picture that future. This may not be an immediate choice, as the current outlook will appear a particular way depending on the thoughts you become entangled with. But as you gain insight, practice being present, and gather self-awareness, you will begin to notice the difference between what is actually happening and the thoughts you are having. Within this space is the opportunity to transcend and ease your suffering.

Confusing pain

People are often confused by their pain experiences. Why does it hurt most of the time today but not yesterday? Or, every time I sit in that chair it hurts, but in another chair, it does not. Or, it was really painful when I was walking yesterday, and today I was fine. It does not seem to make sense to the person or to others, which is where some of the disbelief can come from. We see footballers, for instance, rolling around on the floor clutching their knee, only to be up and running at full tilt a few minutes later.

There are many stories and situations like this, because this is exactly how it is. Pain is contextual and based on what has happened before. So, if I experienced pain for the first time whilst sitting in a particular chair or place, that becomes part of the story, or learning. Next time I go to sit in the same chair, I may be thinking it will hurt, which will influence the likelihood. Even if I am not thinking about it though, subconsciously as a prior experience my systems will anticipate this as a possibility within the overall story of sitting in that chair.

In situations when it does not hurt as expected, we feel that we are doing better than expected. This is important to note and acknowledge as it is evidence for getting better.

Why does pain change?

Pain can and does change. This is because each moment is different. Therefore, our experiences that fill our awareness are ever-changing. It is simply a fact of life. In Buddhism, they talk of impermanence, which makes life possible. No matter how you are feeling right now, it will change.

People are often surprised when their pain changes or appears in different places. There is an expectation that it should be consistent. I then ask, why would it ever be the same? How can anything ever be the same when each moment is new? There are never any 'same' moments. Time is always moving forward.

When you examine your own experience by being present, mindful, or meditating, you find that pain is changeable like all perceptions. Whether it is there or not, the qualities and intensity are dynamic just as are the systems from where pain emerges. We should be more surprised if it were the same. You gain insight into the difference between what is actually happening and the thoughts you are entangled with.

Why is this the case? Why do we expect it to be the same? And why do we often believe that pain is the same when asked how it is? One possible reason is that our sense of self remains the same. It is stable, perhaps to give us some sense of certainty within our existence that is actually full of uncertainty.

The reality is that our perceptions are a constant flow, appearing and disappearing without any bidding or effort on our part. There is no constant, one state. What does and can stay the same is the story we tell ourselves, which is typically an unreliable reporting and assessment of how we are, except for that moment. Our memories are unreliable, and our recall is just good enough, but certainly not definite or even particularly accurate.

This is why we must be careful and skilful with how we interpret our situation, remembering impermanence (see section) as a part of life.

Pain is complex

We are complex, pain is complex. Trying to simplify it often does no justice to the experience or how we can help others or ourselves. However, it does need to be understandable and make sense to the person.

Our knowledge and thinking about pain have moved on enormously over the past 10 years. This is both exciting and hopeful—there is great hope! Through the complexity comes opportunity. Whilst the explanations are more intricate and necessitate some depth, the fact that we can account for varying experiences, test results, and the science of pain is a huge advantage. We are able to bring these elements together to give meaning to your experience.

Pain is part of life. Persistent pain is sometimes called maladaptive or described as something going wrong in the system. I disagree. Having listened to and worked with thousands of people over many years, there is always a reason why pain makes sense in their life. Once you understand that pain is poorly related to the tissues and pathology, and more related to you (the person), your life in the past and now, it begins to make sense. From there, often with skilled guidance, you can find a way forward, shaping a positive future.

Encouragement points and insights

- Understanding your pain is the first step to overcoming your pain.
- Overcoming your pain is an active journey of understanding and learning.
- Pain is complex, but within that complexity, you can understand your experiences and take the opportunities to get better.
- Pain can and does change. This becomes apparent when you examine your own experiences more closely.
- Pain, like all perceptions, varies according to circumstances.
- Pain is a vital part of how we maintain our health and survive.
- You will represent pain to yourself in a unique way dependent on your beliefs, experiences, expectations, and the situation you are in. And because of this, there is possibility and opportunity.

Pain is what the person says it is

There are different definitions of pain, although few capture the essence of the experience like the one by Margo McCaffery (1968): Pain is whatever the experiencing person says it is, existing whenever the experiencing person says it does.

This definition is such a simple and relatable way of describing pain. It has resonated since I was training to be a nurse in the early 1990s but has a longer history. McCaffery was an American pioneering nurse who taught and influenced widely. She wanted nurses and other clinicians to understand the person who was suffering and to be able to help them ease their symptoms and improve their lives. It was not just about defining a subjective experience. You can see why this has been so influential upon me.

Within the language and the approach, you can't fail to see the compassion, a caring concern that one acts upon wisely. There is absolute acknowledgement of the person that in the most modern understanding of pain is the means by which pain is lived—by the person. To try to reduce pain to anything other than the person is somehow trying to reduce the experience, which you cannot. There is no brain scan study, MRI scan, blood test, cell, or receptor on a nerve that can be described as pain. You cannot see pain and to suggest that a result from a test or research study is pain is essentially wrong and missing the point.

Pain is 'whole person': I am or you are in pain. Indeed, it is felt in a particular location, but it is not the body part (location) that is in pain. It is you who is in pain at that moment, the only real moment. McCaffery's definition alludes to this fact, very much leaning towards understanding what it is like for you by listening to what you say. Creating a safe and trusting environment, then, is a key part of helping you describe your pain.

This is not to say that there is no role for tests and studies—just in case you were wondering. Building our knowledge is a vital part of deepening understanding via quality research and performing valid tests. But the results must be put in the light of the human experience. Bringing together the first-person (what it is like for you) and the third-person experience (tests, objective measures) is key. Both are needed and require validation and explanation for the person so that they feel heard and understood.

Mick Thacker and Lorimer Moseley, both physiotherapists and researchers of note, wrote about this back in 2012, pointing out the problem with mereological fallacies: 'the misattribution of a property of the whole being to a single part of that being'. They encouraged the clinical community to consider and incorporate first-person perspectives into their approach to pain by going beyond standard questions to ask about how the person feels, the impact on their life, and the meaning of their pain to them. There are echoes of McCaffery here by being interested in and caring for the person via the questions and subsequent listening required to establish the first-person perspective. Once the clinician knows what it is like for you, then explaining tests and other findings in light of this is the next step.

Reducing pain to anything other than the person means that you can quite simply miss an important aspect of the experience. For example, describing pain as in the brain or because of a particular receptor in the nervous system fails to take into account many of the interrelated dynamics that emerge as pain. Both would be convenient in terms of finding possible treatments because we could look for something that addresses them directly. But this is not how it works as much research has shown. On trying to modify a single factor, the outcomes have been poor. This is because the whole person is not taken into account. Neither is their environment and a multitude of other variables that are put to one side (controlled) in a study.

Again, I emphasise that there is an importance of studies to build the picture. But only in the light of the whole and understanding the limitations. For instance, a study using male rats will only tell us so much about pain in the human being. This is a recognised issue, particularly when trying to learn about pain and gender differences. It goes without saying that humans live different lives to rats, in some respects.

So, what do we need to do? In short, be able to zoom out and in, but then out again to give meaning to your narrative. This we can do by incorporating your experiences with all of the understood science to date. We can bring it together and this creates a strong foundation from where you can move forward.

The International Association for the Study of Pain (IASP) also has a definition: 'An unpleasant sensory and emotional experience associated with, or resembling that associated with, actual or potential tissue damage' (IASP, 2020). Notice something missing?

IASP added six key notes in addition:

- Pain is always a personal experience that is influenced to varying degrees by biological, psychological, and social factors.
- Pain and nociception are different phenomena. Pain cannot be inferred solely from activity in sensory neurons.
- Through their life experiences, individuals learn the concept of pain.
- A person's report of an experience as pain should be respected.
- Although pain usually serves an adaptive role, it may have adverse effects on function and social and psychological well-being.

- Verbal description is only one of several behaviours to express pain; the inability to communicate does not negate the possibility that a human or a nonhuman animal experiences pain.

In the notes, the notion of the person appears but not in the actual definition. Without a person, there cannot be pain, so for me, there is a fundamental issue with the start point. The notes make a substantial difference. The question is whether clinicians take the notes into consideration when working with a person in front of them. A further problem with this definition lies with the focus on damage. We know only too well from both studies and people's experiences that there is absolutely no need for any actual or potential tissue damage, for there to be pain.

Bearing this in mind, I return to McCaffery in 1968. We can put you, the person, right at the heart of our care, listen to what you say (your experiences, beliefs, feelings, insights), consider any results and relevant scientific knowledge, and give meaning to what you are living in your world.

Caring concern is central to working with people who suffer. This is an approach or way of being. A number of professions could fall under the umbrella of caring (the caring professions) in principle, however, it is down to the individual clinician and therapist to embody this way of being. Definitions, models, and schools of thought shape healthcare professionals, as do systems and societies in which they work. But with caring being at the forefront, anything that appears to be a barrier to administering it, should be examined and modified.

The start point for this book is that pain is what you say it is, existing whenever you say it does.

Then onwards to shaping a positive future as defined by you.

Pain truths

There are many messages about pain in society, some of which are outdated or untrue. Unfortunately, many people still feel that they have not been heard or seen with the so-called invisible illnesses. Of course, you cannot see pain or illness per se, but you can see a person who is suffering. Just because pain is not visible, it does not mean that it is not real—it is very real and must be acknowledged.

In this brief section, I have made a series of statements about pain based on what we know in 2023—pain truths for now. I suspect and hope our knowledge will develop so that we can help you more and more skilfully and precisely. Having said that, there's plenty we can do already to help you on your way.

I think this is important because as you read this book and understand all the interrelated dimensions of the pain experience, I want you to know that you are being heard, that I know your pain is real but there are many different ways you can go about easing and transforming your suffering. This is a brief guide and a reminder you can come back to when you want to refresh and sharpen your insights.

I have noticed over the years that the people who do well on their journey are those who take on board the insights and work them into their lives.

In no particular order:

Pain truths

- Pain is what you say it is—a lived experience.
- Pain is always real.
- Pain is a perception.
- Pain is a prediction—or best guess about what is happening for you in your world (context and environment) in this moment
- Pain is personal and unique to you—no one can feel your pain.
- Pain is shaped by your beliefs, past experiences, your attention, expectations, context, and the environment (not individually but rather as they all come together in a circumstance).
- Pain is poorly related to the state of the body tissues (i.e. muscles, joints, discs) or pathology—think about phantom limb pain.
- The body tissues (e.g. discs, joints, muscles, tendons) do not have the ability to produce pain.
- No moment of pain is ever the same, despite how it may appear—impermanence is an important insight into the nature of life. Also, you cannot go backwards. Unless you own a time machine.
- Pain is vital for survival.
- Pain is not in the brain.
- Pain is not a process; it is a lived experience.
- It is you the person that feels pain, not a body part or the brain.
- Pain is embodied—you feel it in your body. But pain is not coming from your body. It is being generated by body systems working together as an ensemble (e.g. nervous, immune, endocrine).

- Pain cannot be seen in any investigation, like hunger or thirst—all are subjective experiences dependent on the person and the situation you are in.
- You cannot reduce pain to anything less than a person in a (their/your) world (you only need to think about your own experience to understand).
- Pain can and does change because it is grounded in your belief system that can be updated in many ways—see the practices and tools section.
- You can understand and overcome your pain. It is challenging and ambitious, but possible.

Some may make sense now. Some may not. Hang in there!

Can pain get better?

This is such an important question. To answer it can be challenging, but I think it is vital that we talk about it and define what is meant by better. Fundamentally, whether you feel better or not can only be determined by you. You decide.

How do you measure it?

There are scales and scores of course. Do they capture your lived experience?

Mostly, you will measure how you are by how you are in that moment: How am I? Current and recent experiences will flavour how you feel you are doing (How am I, and how well am I doing?). This brings bias of course, and being able to zoom out and look at the bigger picture is important. What is the overall trend? What are the circumstances? This gives you a better view. Trying to be objective can be tricky, but it is possible. It is a skill to practice.

The short answer to the question 'can chronic pain get better' is yes. When you examine your own experience more closely, you will see how it is changing. How you are feeling now is not how you will feel; that's impossible, as each moment is different. You feel better sometimes, and worse at other times. It is up and down, like all else in life. Changeable.

Now I will go on to discuss some of the important points. You may feel some discomfort, irritation or resistance when reading what I say. This is normal. When different ideas hit your beliefs, it can evoke a response.

My gentle encouragement is to notice these feelings and acknowledge them—as I do when I am with someone in the clinic or online. Being willing to do this is an important step in transforming your experience. The response is immediate and automatic and hence not something you can control at that moment. However, you can take responsibility and then create a new response.

One of the key ways of overcoming pain is by updating your beliefs. Now you have read the 'What is pain?' section, you understand this. Your beliefs play a role in shaping your actual pain experience. Change beliefs in line with what we know about pain and what you can do to move forward, and the experience of pain changes. If you need to re-read it, then do.

Pain-free?

Many people will set a goal to be pain-free. This is understandable. However, there are some considerations with making pain-free a goal.

Firstly, to be pain-free would be to rid ourselves of an important evolutionary experience and device that protects us. People who are genetically unable to experience any pain sadly do not have long lives (CIP). Secondly, is this realistic considering the circumstances? Thirdly, by wanting to be pain-free, the focus comes immediately back to the pain. With attention and thinking about pain playing a part in shaping the perception, we actually need to be trying to focus on the things we can do to get better. The more we toy with the pain, like poking a snake with a stick, the more we suffer.

So whilst wanting to get rid of the particular pain that is causing suffering (it is important to be precise about this pain rather than pain as a whole) is understandable, to focus on this means you are focusing on the outcome rather than the step to take now. And it is this step now that is you creating the conditions to feel better, sustainably. There is no way to summon a pain-free state. There is no button to press. But you can create the conditions, starting by understanding your pain and how it has become stuck.

As described later in the book, this is not an encouragement to ignore your pain, far from it. You can acknowledge and accept it, both important and be present before practicing ways of transforming pain. To ignore or distract without taking that first step means you are ignoring your own (biological) needs, like thirst or hunger. Maybe sometimes it is necessary to do this for a short time, but generally this is a message that something needs to be done to restore healthy function.

Having said that, I am a firm believer in choosing actions that focus on improving life, and as a (major) part of this journey, easing pain and suffering—

that is the aim, but by focusing on living. How far this will go, no one can say. The future is always uncertain, despite what anyone says. It is by having an uncertain future that life presents possibilities and opportunities—this is a way of representing life to yourself. Pain and life can improve in many different ways depending on your beliefs, openness to possibility, letting go of past history, what you focus on, and your imagination.

It also depends on how you see your life, how much control you feel that you have, and the types of messages you give yourself over and over. What picture are you painting? Because this becomes your reality. But it is not set in stone. You can change your stories. You are free to make this decision. It is not necessarily easy, but it is possible and gets easier. I hope the practices in this book encourage and help you achieve a different story. One that works for you and brings the results you desire.

Some of the ways that people have described getting better include:

- I can do more …
- I enjoy things now …
- I live a full life and deal with the pain when I have to …
- I am back to …
- that particular pain has gone

One of the noticeable changes is the language people use. The focus shifts to what you want and what you can do, which demonstrates a change in your beliefs and expectations. This is the upward spiral as the past ceases to define your future and you are open to possibility and what is available to you. Avoidance that just maintains the fear is replaced by approach as you consciously imagine the future you desire and then step into those shoes.

Updating your beliefs about yourself and your experiences means your thoughts and feelings change and in turn your pain can change as it is grounded in them. This is happening already as you gain new knowledge by reading this book. The resulting behaviours and actions are now different, which they need to be in order to achieve different and better results. There is no other way! Doing the same things and expecting different results is the often-quoted definition of madness, yet as human beings we all fall prey to this trap. Now you are aware, you have the opportunity to take advantage of your potential for transforming your suffering and gaining freedom.

You will have your own unique version of this picture of success.

You can write it down now if you like:

*** my picture of success is:*

To have an impact and to send a strong message to yourself about your picture of success, you need to feel it. Take it beyond a thinking exercise to one that is immersive, using all your senses, makes it much more powerful. Bring the picture to your mind, feel it, see it, taste it, smell it—use all your senses.

Knowing exactly what you are working towards is key. You will look at this in more detail in section 5.

The check in: How am I? What is happening to me right now?

Rating how you are doing is something that you do when people ask, including when you have therapy sessions. You will most likely be monitoring your progress yourself. Have you noticed what you use to decide? Which measures? And importantly, do you take into account how you are feeling when you make this judgement? The state you are in will determine how you think and see the world in that moment. So, if you are suffering, you are more likely to think that you are doing worse than expected. Whereas if you are having a good or better day, you will rate your progress better. This is a completely normal variation. Having this insight helps you understand the dynamic nature of your experiences.

There are other influences on how you report. For instance, who you are speaking to and what you want them to think. You may give people who you are closer to a more accurate description than another person who you don't know very well. In some cases, you may go into more detail about what you are doing and in others you may be brief. Some people I have worked with have found that preparing different scripts for different situations can be helpful. They don't need to be word for word but follow general themes according to the message you want to give.

Measuring how you are over short time periods doesn't necessarily paint a precise picture. Zooming out and looking back over a longer span can give you a more accurate sense of the ups and downs and the overall direction.

How well you are doing relates to how well you expect to be doing and how you expect to be in your life. You could call this your global expectation that incorporates how you are feeling, what you have achieved, and how things are overall for you. This is largely driven by prior experiences and your beliefs about the way things should be for you. When they are not as expected or are not happening with the speed that is expected, you feel as if you are not doing so well. But, of course, this is your own interpretation and perception, which is different from how things actually are in the world. This is certainly the case if you set your expectations too high, find uncertainty challenging or feel that you must be and look a particular way.

In short, there is a world out there and you have your own unique experience or version of the world: a reality and our reality. The latter is shaped by many individual factors and is something we can work with to update our experiences. There is immense power in this possibility when it comes to shaping a positive future.

Setting the bar too high or struggling with uncertainty could be your way. This is not a conscious choice but conditioned, so not your fault. However, you then have the exhausting and stressful job of trying to control the world, situations, and people that you cannot control. There is a continued sense of not doing well because of this fact. To give this up, lose the resistance, and roll with life can seem impossible or perhaps threatening. But this is the way to ease suffering and often pain as instead you focus on what you can control, self-care, and compassion and building health towards a life of freedom.

Gaining insights into your way of being, your beliefs, and your expectations is important alongside understanding pain as a starting point. Then you will come to know why you choose certain actions over others, behave in particular ways, and the reasons for your suffering. It is only by shifting these can you adopt new behaviours that deliver the kinds of results you desire.

When should you start? There's only one moment.

Now.

A question that has kept philosophers busy for many years is a simple one: *Who am I?*

This could be the starting point for you as you gain a new perspective or position from where you see the world. Contemplating this, you come to realise that you are not your thoughts, or your body or your pain. You are the one who hears your thoughts, feels your body, and your pain. This is a very different and empowering position compared to believing that you are those things and being entangled.

We look at your expectations later in the practical section of the book. They are important to know because this is what you think should happen, or is the way you should be, or the way the world should show up. But is it reality? Any mismatch of expectation and reality requires an adjustment of some kind, by changing your expectations and bringing them in line with what is.

Here are some questions you can consider that reveal your expectations of yourself and life:

- What are my expectations of myself? What should I be doing and how?
- What should my life be like? How is my life?
- What should I be achieving? What have I achieved?
- How do I expect to be doing? How well am I actually doing?

What does overcoming pain mean?

You won't be surprised to know now that this is individual and something to clarify at the beginning. Why so? The expectations that you have about how well you think you can recover set the bar. What actually happens for you is measured against this, whether you are thinking about it or not. How well you are doing is registered as a feeling state, which in turn can be considered information that you can use to determine if you are on the right track or not.

We cover this in more detail in the 'Expectations' section. It is tied closely with what you expect of yourself, typically a set of deep-seated beliefs that have been installed previously, which in turn drives the choices you make. The choices you make then deliver a set of results. But are these the ones you want or not?

It starts with knowing and setting your expectations at a level that matches the reality of your situation. This can be hard, especially if we set them high and then become self-critical when they are not met. Getting this right more often than not and making subtle adjustments is an important part of overcoming pain and your well-being.

What do you think about overcoming your pain? What does this look like to you? If you overcome your pain, what does this look like? What would you be doing? Do you believe that you can? These are all important questions.

The types of things people have said to me about overcoming their pain include:

- I am now in control
- The pain does not dominate my life
- I feel free
- I am living a life of possibility
- I rarely feel that pain now

The last comment is noteworthy. The pain they sought help for had eased, which can bring clarity. For instance, once a patient emailed me to say that they had cycled a huge distance and for the first time in a long while, it was the feeling of exercise that hurt and not his hip.

I hope that this gives you a way of thinking about getting better that frames your way forward, using some of the practices in the next sections.

How are you representing your pain?

This is a useful question you can ask yourself.

Now you know that we don't directly experience ourselves or the world. Instead, we have a representation of ourselves and the world shaped by beliefs, expectations, prior experiences, the situation you are in, and more. This can be difficult to take on board as it feels like you are having a direct experience. However, consider that your brain is encased in your skull and therefore does not have access to the world or your body. Instead, your brain receives sensory data and is continually anticipating and predicting the meaning of this information. Somehow, our lived experience emerges from this. Wow!

This being the case, your empowerment emerges from becoming aware of the shaping factors and deciding to focus on those that put you into resourceful states. And update those that do not. This is a skill you can practice.

There are many examples of people being in very tough situations, yet they were able to access their resources to deal with it. I am not saying that this is easy, but it is possible with understanding, self-compassion, and practice. You can do this.

If you represent the pain you are feeling right now in a way that means there is nothing you can do and that it will never end, it will feel a particular way. You are also unlikely to take action because there would be no point. You have no power. This kind of stuckness is common and it is important to emphasise that this is not your fault. You have been and are doing your best, but limiting beliefs that you have accumulated, are constraining your progress.

If you represent the pain you are feeling right now as impermanent, knowing it will change (a life truth), and that there are actions you can take right now, it will feel very different. You will choose certain behaviours and put your full heart into them. There is no definite outcome as you don't know the future, but it makes it much more likely you will succeed. And if you don't get the results you desire, you will try something else, recognising that it takes time. You have the intent to create the best conditions to make it possible for your picture of success to happen. That is what you can do and control.

I hope this helps clarify your current position and gives you hope and the beginnings of the know-how that you will build upon in next sections of this book.

Encouragement points and insights

- Getting better is a personal and individual journey.
- Pain can and does change.
- Setting your expectations is a skill, and a vital one for success.
- Rating your own recovery is affected by the way you are feeling now.
- There are many different ways to measure and acknowledge your success, which is important for getting better.
- You can represent your painful situation (in this moment, the only moment) in different ways: disempowering or resourceful. What position will you take now you have new knowledge and know-how?

Section 5 Starting out

Contents

Clarifying your picture of success

What do you want to achieve? What are the real results that you desire? Can you picture it using your imagination?

Clarifying your picture of success gives you direction. What is it that you are working towards each day? And to be more precise, at this moment, what can you do that is in line with your picture of success?

This is your start point. I encourage you to take your time and think about the types of things you want to be doing, doing more of and re-engaging with now and in time.

Take a blank piece of paper and a pen. Write down all the things that come to mind. Don't limit yourself. Keep going until you can think of no more.

Next, write down why they matter. Why are they important to you? Having reasons is a powerful motivator. You are making decisions based on your values.

Now you can go back and look through your list and choose your top 5. This does not mean that the others are not important. These can be addressed later, as can the how.

What difference would it make to your life if your top 5 were achieved? How would it look? What would you be doing differently? Visualise them and notice how you feel. Where do you feel it in your body? Take a few moments to be aware. This makes it whole, meaning that you are fully immersed in your whole self rather than it being just a thought.

You have been thinking about possibilities. In one sense, life is just about possibility. What can I do? The reason why you may not think like this is because of limiting beliefs that you have accrued through no fault of your own. Think of all the times that you have been told that you can't or won't, especially in your younger years. When you understand that the past does not need to define your future, you begin to feel the freedom that exists. The future is a blank slate because it does not exist and never comes. So, you can fill that blank slate with whatever you want.

You can do this now if you like, and see how it feels.

It doesn't mean that you will achieve all of those things for sure as no one knows the future. But it does mean you will access your resourceful states and take action that makes it much more likely. You will persevere and when you don't get the results you are after, you will try something else. Why? Because the outcome matters to you.

I suggest that you use a journal (see Introduction) and write down your picture(s) of success for daily review. Once you have achieved a result, you can refer to your original list and identify a new one to work towards.

Your picture(s) of success are like islands you are sailing towards on your boat. When you are drifting off course or blown in a different direction by life's inevitable crosswinds or waves (or ups and downs), you can re-establish your direction only by knowing where you are going. Then you use your skills to get back on course. Some days there can be many adjustments as you detect that you are drifting (not feeling so good). In terms of the feeling states that are guiding you, developing your self-awareness and presence helps you to notice the subtleties and nuances for course correction towards your picture of success. Even if it is a long-term goal.

You can ask yourself: Is this a step towards my picture of success?

As some say, you can only score if you know where the goal is.

Your goal is your imagined future. It does not exist right now, but you want it to manifest by way of the conditions you create through the decisions that you make each day. That's you in the driving seat, empowered and focusing on what you can control.

If you like, you can start here.

My picture(s) of success are:

1.

2.

3.

4.

5.

Your strengths

Everyone has strengths. They bring us success when we play to them, over our weaknesses. We all have these too. Mike Pegg (2012) consistently makes the point that we can build on our strengths and manage the consequences of our weaknesses to achieve on-going success. This is also my encouragement to you.

It is useful to be aware of our own strengths, making a list of the top 3—more if you like. You have many! One way of doing this is by thinking of an example of when you were successful. What were you doing? How did you go about the task? How was it that you achieved your desired results? Which strengths did you use? Picture this situation noticing the images, your inner language, and how it feels. Notice your change in state.

This is also useful material for your journal that can be reflected upon and used practically.

A simple daily habit is to choose a strength and each day you practice. For example, perseverance could be a strength you have identified from a prior success. You can think about how you kept going until you delivered. What did you do exactly, and how can you repeat that now, in this situation? Again, feel it, taking the practice beyond a thought exercise into a lived experience.

You can complete the following practice:

A time when I was successful was:

The strengths I used to be successful were:

1.

2.

3.

The ways I can use these strengths now are:

1.

2.

3.

Your values: What matters to you?

Your values are the important principles that you live by. Your daily decisions depend upon the values that have been instilled in you and those you choose to adopt.

You have been conditioned to believe certain things about yourself and the world. This comes from your upbringing, education, society, culture, experiences, and realisations. You don't have a choice in how much of this turns up in your life. You didn't choose to be you, to have your mind, or to even exist! But here you are. Having this insight helps you realise a life truth, but then importantly, know that you can take responsibility for your life and how you go about things.

What matters to you will impact how you prioritise. For instance, if you believe that working hard is important, you will decide to do this over something else that is less significant in your eyes. Another person could view this the other way round.

When it comes to health, people know this is important. Yet not everyone will make decisions based on health being a priority. In reality, health is arguably one of the most important aspects of your life (see next section). All else stems from being and feeling healthy and well. It is in these states that you can do your best, especially when it comes to the challenge of overcoming pain.

One of the reasons for being clear on your values and living by them is that you will be motivated to take action in line with your picture(s) of success. When you know your 'why', you will almost certainly find it easier to work out the how because it matters to you.

When I ask people to name their top three values, often they say their work, family, and health. Whilst these seem obvious, they are not actually living this way. Instead, they are swayed and distracted by modern living, social messages, and influences. There is strong encouragement to opt for a quick fix or short-term pleasure rather than do the necessary work to understand themselves, the situation and take the steps towards transformation.

For example, it is typically considered acceptable and permissive for people to have a drink to deal with stress rather than face and deal with the reasons for the stress. Further, you can go for a cigarette break during the day at work, but you would get a less supportive response to the announcement that you are going outside to take some air or to practice a yoga pose.

The rewards for the quick fixes feel good and are immediate, hence the appeal. Healthy actions, however, take time and repetition over months and years. In fact, all of the important things in life require consistent practice throughout our lives: loving relationships, health, and purpose. Interestingly, many of these are not strictly measurable as they are felt by the individual subjectively. Giving them a score out of ten captures none of the richness of the actual experience that only the individual can feel.

Quick and cheap fixes litter our society. There are many offerings and promises using overt marketing to grab your attention. They are part of our day-to-day experience of social media, advertising, and conversation—being asked, 'Have you tried?' It is up to you to decide whether there is value in what is being offered, which is not easy to navigate with convincing marketing. If it seems too good to be true, it probably is. Chronic pain is complex and dynamic. To simplify it moves away from reality and credible ways forward.

You may have expected your pain and symptoms to get better quickly, or within a certain timeline, having had some treatment or taking medication. Sometimes things do improve quickly, but sometimes they don't. Many people get stuck, which is illustrated by the huge numbers suffering persistent pain across the globe—some 20% of the population.

You want to be back doing all the things you were doing. This appears to be reasonable and is often possible after an injury. Many people do recover and resume their valued activities. This takes time. The body's time, not yours! It may be longer than you want, but the time is what you need together with creating the right conditions. When you understand the timelines, you can set your expectations at the right level. Failing to meet incorrect expectations is one way we contribute to the development of chronicity. More on the art and skill of setting expectations later—it's an important one.

When you have your (top) values at the forefront of your thinking, you make better decisions in line with these manifesting in your life. You create the conditions for health and well-being to emerge. When you let your values slide, there can be ill effects that persist. Essentially, by putting health and other important things on the back burner, we are creating the conditions for ill health, in part by the stress caused by a mismatch of values and your lived life.

What would this look like? Minimal exercise and activity, sedentary lifestyle, poor diet, lack of sleep (most people need 7–8 hours) and persistent stress (contributed to by a lack of balancing factors) are some of the unsurprising factors. So, if we know this, how does it happen? Life and how we get caught up is what happens to us.

No one does it on purpose. Their circumstances, abilities, and choices are such that you are doing the best you can to cope. I always assume that someone else in the same situation would make similar choices. We could all be there.

I have seen a number of people who have not recovered from injuries or surgery as expected due in part to this mismatch of values within their life.

The good news is that there is a way out. It is not necessarily easy, but it is possible to understand and face the challenge, before moving forward in a positive way. That is the message of this book.

Thinking about your values now, what are your top 3? You can write them down below to make them clear in your thinking to drive your actions.

Bringing them to your awareness, you can now start making decisions consistently with your values in mind. In particular, this is useful when designing your way forward. Motivating yourself to practice each day becomes a value-based decision. It matters to you. When you have a good reason, you will always find a way.

When you tie this with the reward from taking a positive action in line with your picture of success and focusing on the process over the prize, successes come frequently. Little wins are available to you when you make this your way and acknowledge them. This is the basis for skilfully managing your expectations to meet the reality of your current situation, remembering that how things are now are not how they will be. In turn, this is you shaping your perceptions and experiences of the world and yourself in ways that you want. This is what you can control.

My top 3 values are:

1.
2.
3.

You may like to take a blank piece of paper and write out all your values, before narrowing them down to your top 3.

Your beliefs about pain

There is a way you are thinking about your pain right now based on your belief system. In particular, your higher beliefs are playing out as your experience of pain. If you are having pain experiences over and over (not the same as they cannot be the same, but similar), there is a stuckness in your body systems, which are not updating. This results in similar predictions, pain, in certain situations.

Getting unstuck, then, needs an examination of your beliefs and then an update, installing some new ones based on new understanding and experiences that you curate and create with guidance and encouragement (the essence of Pain Coaching). The practices and tools are the ways you can do this together with a new level of awareness, presence, and self-compassion.

The beliefs you have about your pain are formed when you are young and are shaped throughout your life. We have painful experiences of falling, grazing, sore throats, and other common childhood illnesses and incidents. They are training your body systems that protect you and organise healing. You have an incredible ability to heal without having to consciously do anything. It just happens for you. However, this process will be more effective if you are creating the best conditions by looking after yourself and practicing self-compassion.

There is no reason why you would necessarily know this, although you experience the workings of your body systems each day as a matter of feelings, thoughts, and emotions. They are all information and a guide as to how you are doing right now.

Right now, then, you have a belief and a way of thinking about injuries and pain, based on what has happened to you in the past. This is learning and conditioning in action.

Commonly, the belief is that you injure yourself, it hurts, you look after yourself how and if you can, or you seek help if you think you can't. As a child, you may have been soothed by your parent or someone else. You could have been taken to a doctor who would ask a few questions, often to your parent, then make a suggestion as to what should be done. Often you would leave the office clutching a prescription that you take to the local chemist, collect your medication, start taking the pills and sure enough, you start to feel better.

This is a powerful medical model. A series of clear steps that lead to recovery. I have had this experience, and I would imagine that you have too. And it shapes how we think things will work in the (imagined) future. So, with this sequence embedded, some years later, you injure yourself, head to the doctor, he/she asks some questions, you answer, he/she gives you a prescription, you go to the chemist to collect your medication, you take the pills and you don't get better. Now what? Your expectations and the reality have shifted. The model did not work as you expected or wanted. Why?

Because this is an oversimplified model that does not consider the big picture and all the circumstances that are relevant for pain and injury. Or the fact that pain and injury are poorly related.

At the time, you don't realise your world view is misaligned with reality because you don't have the knowledge available to you—not your fault. In many cases, this view takes the form of a passive approach to getting better. Something happens to you, you seek help, and someone else makes you better via their actions. These are the passive treatments when methods are applied to you: for example, massage, acupuncture, and manipulation. Essentially, someone is fixing you and you may search for someone to fix you because this is your belief based on what you have experienced before. And before, it may have helped, or so you believe. So, it makes sense to do it again. But then if it doesn't work.

Then what do you think? The therapy doesn't work? The therapist is no good? Does it occur to you that getting better is a proactive process that you must undertake? Yes, treatments may play a role in you feeling better in the short term. However, sustained recovery is about you consistently creating the conditions for your body systems to return to day-to-day healthy functioning, considering the circumstances.

The idea of fixing people is on both sides of the table. Much healthcare training comes under the guise of fixing patients—they come along with particular problems that we need to fix.

Just as the childhood visit to the doctor started with a brief question and answer session with varying degrees of compassion, this is what I expect now. Although part of me may feel that I need something else as well. Perhaps an opportunity to describe how I feel about what has happened and how it is affecting me.

So, if there is no fixing to be done, what is the right course of action?

Before answering this question, we can pause to think about your existing beliefs about your pain. This will reveal your position. You may notice how your views are wrapped up with those of your gender, culture, and society in which you live. Messages you have received by parents, within schooling, other caregivers, society at large, or your faith, will all play a role here, not just in your thinking, but in your actual experience of pain. Or as I will refer to it, your perception of pain (see 'What is pain?' for a review).

Get on with it, dust yourself off, you're fine, man up, grow up and more are all words you may have heard at some point. Either directed at yourself or someone close by. The implication is that you should be able to deal with the situation, cope, and move on. If not, somehow you are weak. Of course, this is incorrect and only based on wrong thinking that has been imprinted on the person delivering the message.

Often delivered to children by adults, many children will not have such skills. Because they are children. The limitation sits firmly with the adult whose weakness is revealed by their words and actions as a way of making themselves feel better.

I dwell on this only to make the point that the beliefs of others play such an important role in shaping ours. Whilst I hope you have not had this experience, many do. And this needs to change, which I feel is as we evolve our understanding of pain. A slow process, but I see it happening together with an openness to new knowledge that is emerging and the basis of this work.

One of the most common beliefs about pain that is wrong is that pain and injury are the same or well-related. In fact, we have known that this relationship is fragile for many years. Pat Wall, arguably the founder of modern pain science together with Ron Melzack, wrote about this in a famous paper in 1979:

> *'Pain is better classified as an awareness of a need-state than as a sensation. It serves more to promote healing than to avoid injury. It has more in common with the phenomena of hunger and thirst than it has with seeing or hearing.'*

Here we are in 2023 with most people still thinking incorrectly about pain. Why does this matter?

It matters because if you do not understand pain, it is very easy to go down the wrong path. Sometimes you can do this and it turns out reasonably well, although often it means you carry incorrect beliefs forward to the next time. Of course, these beliefs do not feel as if they are wrong! In fact, the exact opposite.

The existing belief that pain and injury are similar or well-related can be built upon when we are exposed to the predominant biomedical model. Essentially, this model is the basis of modern medicine, when you look for a cause of pain and symptoms in the body, or the end-organ. The search is on for an injury, a pathology, or a disease that can be identified and then treated. In our world, this makes sense. It does so because it fits with our belief system that has been constructed throughout our lives.

But as you know now, the biomedical model does not answer all the questions that we have about pain. We need a different model that is able to explain phantom limb pain, pain when there is no injury or pathology, the varying pain perceptions that people describe, and how things get better. It is a model such as predictive processing that does appear to be able to do this, and where we must go with our inquiry and understanding to address the problem of pain, which is vast and global.

Under normal conditions, if we injure ourselves, we expect it to hurt somewhat. The type of experience we have and how intensity varies. Everyone will have their own perception and sense of what it is like to be in pain. Each pain experience is unique, each moment. This appears to confirm ideas that pain and injury have a one-for-one relationship. Yet the close examination of one's experience, which we rarely do unless you are a meditator, reveals something different.

Your experiences are dynamic. Each moment is fundamentally different and never the same. Think about when you tell yourself that something is the same. It cannot be. The only thing that is the same is the story you tell yourself. Life is only possible because each moment is different and because time flows (at seemingly different speeds depending on the circumstance—another trick of perception). This is the concept of impermanence, which makes life possible.

Stepping back you will notice that the things you tell yourself over and over can become your truth and reality. Yet this may not be what is actually happening. There are and can be mismatches. The experiences that we have are not direct representations of ourselves and the world. They are your brain's best guesses, which are usually good enough.

Yet you can get stuck on certain beliefs. And it seems that around pain, this is often true. Perhaps because pain is arguably tied up in protection and survival, certain danger signals are afforded greater priority, and the brain's job is to ensure you continue living, it means that you hold on tight to your views. Yet if they are wrong, it can result in decisions being made that are not in line with what you want to achieve.

An important question beyond an exploration of existing beliefs is: how open you are to other explanations for your pain? And if not, why not? Why is there a stickiness or rigidity? These are all important areas to understand and develop, otherwise they could be holding you back from reaching your potential.

This is illustrated by the person who believes that each time they experience their pain they are doing something harmful or damaging. Understandably, this belief would cause them to decide to reduce their activity or avoid certain movements. For instance, back pain and bending.

There has been much said and written about bending our backs. Essentially the encouragement or sometimes with firm orders, we are told not to bend because it is bad for our backs. Think of all the pictures that show a figure slightly stooped, clutching their back. Others with a person bending over, covered with a big red cross, perhaps with words underneath, don't or wrong.

I have met many people suffering persistent low back pain who have limited their movements for years. On top they have added a lot of sucking in of their abdominal muscles and sometimes their buttocks. Each time they go to move, they pull it all in and tensing up. This becomes their way of protecting themselves.

Repeated anticipation of movements and actual movements in this guarded, tense way builds just that for the future. You start to expect to move this way consciously and subconsciously, and sure enough it becomes your way of bending. It is understandable why you would continue and to defend this as a way that works for you despite the cost (e.g. more energy, reinforcing protection rather than free movement). And if it works for you, why change? Plus, any evidence that supports another way can be seen as threatening or wrong.

So somehow, to move forward in a healthy direction, we need to reposition ourselves, but often without being told directly—no one likes being told what to do! Much better is when you come up with the plan based on a conversation about change. You challenge your own belief because it is important to you to improve your life by expanding your choices. Whilst your limited back movements and way of moving allow you to feel safe, it does not permit you to live the life you want. This is a value-based decision (see Your values).

By shining a light on your belief, you can create an opportunity to make a change. It can feel worrying, evoking strong emotions sometimes, but here is your chance to evolve and get better even though in the short term it can feel very different. A part of you may even be saying that what you are now doing is wrong. It requires courage and perseverance with the right kind of support and encouragement. In my view, this is the essence of good therapy.

Limiting the bending of a tense back for a long period of time will have its inevitable consequences on both the health of the tissues and the experience of what it is like. Remember that the two do not have to match exactly. For example, a study (Stanton et al., 2017) showed that there was a difference between the actual and perceived stiffness of the back tissues. The authors argued that the reason for the perception was to motivate the person to move more. That makes sense when you consider the importance of movement. There is not much you can achieve without movement, said Karl Friston.

I hope you can see the importance of examining your beliefs, having conversations based on what we understand and know from the science and then experimenting with something new. But grounded in knowledge and wisdom, surrounded with compassion and care, and exacted with skill and determination to actively make things better.

You can do this exercise to help clarify your current position.

My existing beliefs about pain:

What is pain?

Why am I in pain?

What causes my pain?

In the case of chronic pain, why has it continued?

How willing am I to update my beliefs about my pain?

How do I feel when I am presented with different facts about pain?

What really matters to me?

What action can I take now?

There are no right and wrong answers, just your own honest ones. This is for you to make some discoveries that may be uncomfortable at times, but also enlightening and a way forward.

Your decisions and what we then do are based on our beliefs. To create a new way forward, you need to be aware of what you are doing now and why (what is driving it from underneath), what works for you in the long term (towards our pictures of success), and where you need help and guidance. Through this process you will be able to make better and best decisions more often, thereby delivering success and the results you desire.

Once you have read the book and extracted the knowledge and practical tools, you can review your beliefs on pain once more. But as the Buddha said, do not believe anything simply because you have heard it. Instead, observe and analyse your own experiences and see what benefits you and those around you. So, don't believe me. Come to your own conclusions by exploring your own life, way of being and discover what works for you.

Mike Pegg, pioneer of strengths-based coaching, has said to me and others, take the best and leave the rest. Wise words.

Encouragement points

- Becoming aware of your beliefs about pain helps you understand the choices you are making
- Your beliefs about your pain are shaping your very experience of pain
- Clarifying whether your beliefs match what is currently known about pain allows you to update and move on
- Which beliefs that you hold about your pain are helping you achieve your picture of success?
- Which are not?

Getting better

We have our own ideas about getting better. When you think about getting better, what does it look like? What would you be doing differently if you were better? These are usually your picture(s) of success.

Essentially, getting better is all about the future, which is imagined. You can continually strive to get better at certain skills or being a better person. There is much encouragement to do so. The media, bookshelves, educational institutions, governments, parents, and friends can all encourage you to do better with your lives. Some try to show you how.

Why does this matter? It matters if the way things are right now don't feel good or right. Certainly, when the person suffers persistent pain, they want something better. You will have some ideas about how that life would be for you, dreaming of it, hoping for it, but often unsure how to go about it.

There can be differences between how the person views getting better and how the clinician sees it. Somehow there needs to be a meeting point, although I would argue that the person in pain defines getting better. They are at the centre whilst the clinician listens, guides, and encourages.

The importance of clarifying your picture of success and why it matters is emphasised here. This is the starting point, knowing where you are heading. Then we must devise the steps to get there, recognising that it is in the distance yet possible to get there in time. I encourage a focus on process over prize because to focus on the latter means you are not present or taking the action that you could be right now to go in that very direction. To be present, self-aware, and choosing the best action now are key ingredients for success. This will be emphasised in the practical part of the book (see Practices and tools section).

The types of things people have told me about their experiences of getting better vary enormously. Much of the feeling of achievement rests on where the person sets the bar.

If we think getting better and being successful is being pain-free (in the imagined future), there is repeated disappointment and often a sense of failure. The self-critic can also chime in at this point making things worse. In this case, there is a focus on the prize over the process. Realising that the prize does not materialise by focusing on it and thinking about it helps to re-orientate on the action I can take now to create the right conditions to get better. This is a skill as we tend to become caught up in, wanting something other than what is happening right now.

Another way is to consider getting better as a process and a series of daily mini steps, each of which are successes in themselves. You can then feel good about what you are doing along the way, motivating further action in the right direction. It is the consistent accumulation of such actions that creates the conditions for a better and positive future.

One challenge arises from the fact that every day is not payday. Or put another way, you sow the seeds today, but you won't be eating the fruit. As I have pointed out elsewhere, building wellness (a significant part of getting better) is a long game when you act now for a healthier future. You clean your teeth today for future oral health—and fresh breath now of course. Accepting this as true relieves the pressure of expecting, hoping, and wanting something to manifest immediately. This is not helped by the many things in life we can get now or very soon—for example, download a song or a book, order a pizza, same day delivery.

Beyond what getting better looks like to you, there's the how. How do you think that you will get better? What resources do you already have? Are they working? What help do you need? Usually people come along to see me with some questions but are open to the ideas that I have to share on how to move forward. Some people have pre-existing ideas and tell me what they need. All of these are respected and discussed before agreeing a way forward. There is a togetherness, a collaboration, but led by the person. This is their life.

To you the reader, this is your life and you want it to be different and better in specific ways.

A reasonable question to the clinician is, how will your treatment, approach and methods help me to get better? The clinician should of course be equipped to answer. They will be able to answer this fully if they are a pain specialist.

What is a pain specialist?

This is someone who has the specialist knowledge and skills required to help a person to ease their suffering caused by their pain. This includes the art of being with someone, creating a safe space, being present and listening deeply, empathising, and offering guidance at the right time. This is your journey.

There is no one profession adequately trained at a basic level. Instead, it is an accumulation of specific knowledge drawn from many fields, skills, and the wisdom needed to use them.

True pain specialists can be physiotherapists, nurses, doctors, psychologists, or other healthcare professionals, each offering I think it is always sensible to look at the background of the clinician or therapist you are thinking of working with, to make sure that they are suitable.

Each clinician will have their approach based upon a range of models and experiences. There is no one way, but there are ways that are better suited to you and your needs. The facts about pain and pain science remain the same of course. But the practices, tools and exercises can be nuanced according to the lens through which the clinician looks. My hope is that the primary lens that is used sees a person with strengths and potential to shape a positive future.

Once the approach is established and understood, the picture of success clarified, expectations set at the right level (this is changeable), then the quest for relief, re-connection (with what matters), and recovery can begin. The focus becomes squarely on the best course of action right now, but always in line with the picture of success or the particular goal that is being worked towards. The practice of 'nudging' helps us to remain on course because life will push us in different directions. Sometimes very subtly and other times brutally, with everything else in between.

Now you may like to consider what getting better means to you.

What is getting better? What do I mean by this?

What does getting better look like?

How would my life be different?

Do I believe that this vision is attainable? Am I being realistic?

What do I need to help me be successful in getting better?

Similar to gaining insights into your beliefs that underpin decisions, this will enable you to understand what you view as the end point, how you will get there, and with what kind of help. This knowledge is entirely practical as it guides your decisions. You can delve back into your beliefs and insights at any time to recalibrate and hence keep the desired direction. Repeating these exercises at certain points can be revealing and helpful in this regard.

Following a path to getting better is a choice of action. Only you can decide to use tools and practices in order to shape something more desirable. Only you can take the chosen action and determine the outcome, which reveals itself at different points. We often look for cause and effect, yet in reality this is difficult to determine. Whilst you may do something and it appears that a certain result arises, there are so many unseen and unknown variables in your biology and in the world, that it is impossible to say that A definitely led to B. Being able to zoom out and take a wider perspective is important.

This is not to say that there is no relationship. If I take a hammer and hit my finger, there is a fairly clear relationship between what I did and then feeling something as a consequence. What I feel, however, will vary within a particular context. The way I respond will also be determined by the situation I am in. If I were demonstrating the technique and felt some embarrassment or shame (they are different) having made the mistake, this will undoubtedly affect my pain perception. There are many other social modulating factors together with expectations and prior experiences that shape what it is like for me at that moment. It is certainly not just about danger signals being transmitted from the nerves in my finger to the spinal cord and brain. Each moment we live is being shaped by a huge range of factors, mostly unknown to us at the time.

To some this may sound like you don't have much control. You do have control over certain things, but not perhaps in the way you think. One of the key ways of dealing with the unknowns and uncertainties in life is to be consistent with healthy habits that will bear the fruit of wellness in time. Of course, this needs trust in the process and knowlegde from studies and lived experiences (people's stories). Naturally, these must be judiciously considered in the light of facts. Although even facts may be updated in time.

Making things better appears to be a natural urge. In this context, we are talking about suffering persistent pain and getting better. But this is not separate from the rest of your life, your ambitions, desires, hopes, and dreams. The pain may seem like it is in the way of these and if only it would go away, then I could live the life I so desire. On this, I have a suggestion based on many years of working with people suffering from pain and other ailments who are waiting for this magical moment. This moment is thought to be a possibility by the promises of some who claim to be able to cure you with pills, injections, and other remedies. Most probably take a more considered view that their offerings are part of the help you need.

On the basis that you are reading on, I assume you are ready for what I have to share with you, which I hope and know some people are already doing. Perhaps you.

Now, I ask you to bear with me as I describe it. Read it thoroughly, noting your responses—aha moments, resistance, or something else. Then sit back. It may seem overwhelming or exciting. Each person will react or respond in their own way. You will have yours. I know this, but we are shining the light on your beliefs. But it is this you need for transformation to something better. So, hang in there.

Here we go.

It is simply to focus on living your best life now. In this moment, the only moment.

You need to understand and bear in mind this is dynamic and complex. In other words, how you are now is not how you will be, whatever you choose to do. But let's give it a direction towards what you want. You are constantly changing despite the static sense of self—you feel like you, and still do. So, instead of waiting for someone or something to take the pain away so you can live again, you decide to live to overcome the pain.

Pain rents space. And the less you are connected with what matters and engaged in doing things you love and need to do, the more impacting the pain because it can rent more and more space. You can only pay attention to one thing at a time. The person suffering persistent pain is living many moments filled with pain. There are other moments, but on a 'bad day' (you can call this something else—see Talking to yourself), there are many of the pain-filled ones.

On a better day, there are longer gaps between. You want more of that and to widen those gaps by filling your days with things you want to do in the best way you can considering the current (but not permanent) circumstances.

This may sound easy, but I know it is not. It is challenging, but possible. There are many ways to go about organising your day and ensuring that you are self-caring throughout. I will get into many of those ways in the Practices and Tools section.

A framework to use

The Pain Coaching framework has four main and overlapping themes. They are designed to keep you pointing to the right direction: your picture of success.

Proactive theme (habits)

These are your practices, tools, and strategies that you use each day, working towards the future you and life that you desire. I sometimes call them your daily pillars—actions you definitely take. Steps towards your picture of success that are integrated into your day. Like cleaning your teeth.

This is all about working on existing habits that deliver results, plus adding new ones that address particular factors. For example, the skills of being well that seek to build your wellness, step by step each day. You can think of this akin to cleaning your teeth. Some of these you seek to cement into your routine as practices that are shaping your future. Each time you practice is another step in the right direction.

You will also have some habits that you use less frequently but are an important part of your life. Talking to friends, certain types of exercise (e.g. classes), or groups you attend maybe once a week or month. These things matter and you want to reconnect with them or do more.

Skilful responses to challenging moments

There will be ups and downs. Getting better and making changes is not a linear process. Rather than a straight, smooth pathway, it is more a winding road, with hills and sometimes potholes. In time, you can come to understand that these challenging moments are actually learning opportunities, meaning that you can do it better next time and so on. This is a more productive way of representing a situation that does not fit with your expectations or preferences.

The truth of the matter is that life happens. Life happens regardless of what you or anyone likes or dislikes. That is not the point. The point is that simply life happens and you can be present and handle or enjoy whatever is happening right now.

You can learn and develop many skills that you use to stay on, or get back on track. By learning to 'apply the brakes' and self-soothe, you can lessen the impact. With these skills and practices at hand, plus periodising your days to achieve a balance of activity and rest/recovery, you can navigate your way forward with awareness and increasing confidence. If you think about this, you will see that this is how peak performers work to be successful. You can do the same.

The skills of being well

These are skills and strategies that water the seeds of well-being in you. There are many to choose from as part of your consistent practice to create the best conditions. This is what you can control. Examples include diet, sleep, exercise, communication (with self and others), movement, awareness, connection with other people, and purpose. There are others, and importantly they are tailored to your needs and in support of your work towards your picture(s) of success. Notice that this theme is about focusing on what you want—well-being.

Life skills—how to live your life the best way, including all the day to day activities you want and must do, or work towards doing. This is considering your circumstances and that how things are now is not how they will be because they are ever-changing.

The bulk of your time is spent living your life according to the current circumstances and opportunities. Your practice will take a certain amount of time. Then there is the rest of the day: How many hours are you awake? This time needs to be managed so as to stay on track.

Often when suffering chronic pain, the range of choices and possibilities narrows. Expanding them is one of the goals, together with finding the best way to do so by learning new skills and reconnecting with what matters, bit by bit. In other words, increasingly filling your time with meaningful activities, which is a key strategy. Why? Because it means less room for the pain to rent, and the thoughts about it.

The overlap between these themes is where certain practices perform different roles. Some that are calming and soothing at times of suffering can also be used as daily skills of being well to tone down sensitive body systems and bring online calmer feelings. You can practice these at regular times so that when you need them, you apply them with increasing skill. There is plenty of low-hanging fruit each day to practice dealing with moments of frustration, irritation, anxiety, and discomfort.

Depending on your needs, you will choose those that are most useful for both means. By learning to be more present and self-aware, this becomes easier. Like a craftsman selecting the right tool for the job in front of him or her or an artist choosing the right brush. You are that artist.

What about pain relief? Where does that come into it?

The first insight is that you only need to manage and ease your pain when it is present. A number of the skills are about changing your state, which changes your experience. Because they are skills, each time you practice, you can get a little better.

The second insight is that as you reconnect with what matters in your life and fill your time with meaning and purpose, together with self-caring strategies becoming habitual, there is less likelihood of pain appearing in the first place. Remember that your body systems are generating pain as a best guess to explain your current circumstances (your lived world), but also all your other experiences. So, when you shift your intent, focus, and actions, you begin to gather new sense data to update the predictions, and hence your experiences.

This is what you are doing anyway but now with a direction, your picture(s) of success, to live your best life in your own way.

Pain Coaching

This is a way of being with someone suffering from chronic pain. Driven by compassion, a caring concern to help with guidance, support, and encouragement, Pain Coaching is both person-first and whole person in its philosophy. This stems from my nursing days when the care models and ways of working were reflected in this way. It is also a way of being with yourself. After all, you coach yourself more than anyone else.

Anyone can be a pain coach. It is an umbrella term that encompasses a range of different ways of helping. Some key elements are understanding pain, the ability to create a safe environment, and the ability to listen deeply and empathetically. At the right time, advice is given.

In my view, as clinicians and therapists, we are carers and sharers. We care for people professionally, but importantly, in a human and authentic way. Then we share ways that you can improve your life when you are ready to put them into practice.

One of the aims is to give you, the person, the knowledge, skills, and wisdom to be your own 'self-coach'. This is when you are able to encourage yourself to make clear and best decisions. It includes the type of questions you ask yourself and the language you use. You become a self-directed Pain Coach.

Encouragement points

- When designing your way forward, think about your needs and challenges. Then you can choose different practices and tools to help you.
- Whilst you can be coached by someone else, ultimately you are your own coach (see Self-coaching section). How will you coach yourself? What voice will you use to encourage and motivate? What is your tone and intent?
- Some daily practices (habits) are the steps you are taking proactively towards your picture of success. Other tools are your skilful ways of dealing with challenging moments. You need both.

Self-coaching: Making the difference in your world

You have the freedom to choose your approach and what you do at any given moment. You can set out your intent and your standard. There is something you need to become aware of and deal with though. You could call these automatic thoughts. The ones that just appear. The chatter. The commentator.

And whilst you cannot stop these thoughts coming, like you can't stop the tide coming in, you can get to know your mind (it's different parts and what they say). Bringing this awareness means you can simply let the chatter be without any interference. You are disentangled from these thoughts and they pass. You let them go rather than holding on. It is the holding on that causes us problems. More on this in the practical section. This is a vital skill on the route to freedom from suffering.

This is a double-edged sword because it is up to you, the individual person, to take responsibility and shape your positive future. Whilst some people feel empowered, others are daunted and would rather someone else make them better. There is no blame attached to this because either way, your current position is not your fault. You did not choose your mind or way of thinking. You did not even choose to be you! You have been doing your best with the resources you have. But to start making a difference, this must be realised.

You may need guidance, support, and encouragement from skilled clinicians and therapists. In my opinion, we all need a coach and mentor. There is also a key role for other people around: family and friends. You will be influenced by the people close by. Notice how you behave with different people. Sometimes you want to fit in and make compromises. Other times you want to stand out. You listen to some people, taking on board what they say without question. Others you dismiss. Why?

Much will relate to the values that have been imprinted on you through your life as previously explained. The question is whether they are leading to behaviours that are resulting in the outcomes you want, or not? If not, you can update them. What works you continue with, and the rest is left, replacing them with new skills and practices. Life is continuous and impermanent. What you needed then may not be what you need now. And the way things are now is not how they will be in the future. The future is a blank slate of course. No one knows the future. It is uncertain, which means we need to be comfortable with uncertainty to ride the waves of life.

The idea that we can be fixed is common and inherent in many people's thinking. This is the model you have been shown and one we have all experienced. It is a linear model: something feels wrong, we seek help (e.g. GP), we are told what it is (a diagnosis), someone else does something (given a pill or some kind of treatment) and we get better. Sounds good. But the reality is far more complex. There are innumerable variables, many of which we cannot account for. Now that you have read about pain (see 'What is pain?'), you will have an understanding of the complexity. A simple cause and effect is not what actually happens.

So, considering the complexity and the unknowns, what can you focus on? What can you control? This goes back to the first line of this section. You can choose your approach (see 'Your approach') and think about, and act upon the things you can control, consistently. This I call self-coaching.

Just as I coach you by listening, seeing the circumstances, thinking about the bigger picture and your picture of success and recommending the next best step, you do the same. The moment to moment decisions you make in line with your expectations govern the outcomes or results you achieve. But, just to make things a little more complicated, some types of pain experiences emerge at different time points.

In other words, there is not an immediate stimulus-response relationship. You do something on a given day but do not feel the effects for hours, days, weeks or even months—the biological reasons for this are well understood. You should understand them too, so that you know what is happening when you have certain types of experience (see What is pain?). It could appear to make it difficult to work out what has happened and to choose the best action. However, what it really calls for, is the need to be consistent with our practices as a means to move in a desirable direction. This alongside knowing that you have not done anything wrong per se.

Just as a coach would look at situations that have arisen and you have handled them, you can do this yourself. I encourage people to study their own successes in the main: What has gone well? How were you successful? What principles did you follow? How can you follow them again and build onwards? This is the essence of strength-based coaching (Pegg, 2012).

You can also look at the challenging moments to see what you did and think about what worked and what did not. Learning from past experiences is something we can choose to do. This changes the context of all the situations you face. They can be deemed successful or learning opportunities—the obstacle becomes the opportunity. Now, this is not to say that you want to experience pain in order to learn, or that it is no longer an unpleasant feeling.

But, changing your position on how you think about what has happened and what you do has an impact on your pain experience. You now know that pain experiences are predicted, or best guesses about what is happening right now for you in your world. This is flavoured by the context: where you are, what you are doing, what you have done in this situation before, other prior experiences, expectations, attention, your mood, your thinking, who you are with, the opportunities in the environment, and more. Whilst this is far more complicated than the linear ideas about pain (biomedical), it is the truth about pain (and other perceptions), and importantly, it offers you many ways to take steps towards valued life goals.

Coaching is largely about communication. Who do you talk to most often? Yourself of course! And how do you talk to yourself? What language do you use? Tone? You are responding to this all the time. This is why developing self-awareness matters. You can start to realise how you talk to yourself, the kinds of things you are saying, and the types of responses you are experiencing. I would like to add here, coming through the compassionate lens, that there is no blame attached to the way you think. I will repeat this message often. You did not choose your mind, or to be you even. This is the starting point, before taking responsibility and thinking about better ways forward.

As an example, there can be a part of you that has unrealistic expectations. This results in setting goals that are unachievable, which of course you fail to fulfil. Then the self-critic makes various comments in a particular voice. Or another part of you says that what you are doing is not working. These are strong messages and utterly compelling. You are not choosing to say these things, they just seem to appear and grab us. The problem lies in listening and acting upon them without looking at a balanced view, or seeing that the initial issue was setting the wrong goal.

During a flare up (an increase in symptoms—which is part of the journey), people can start to think that the techniques and tools they are using are not working. When you understand that flare ups are normal (not pleasant) and usually unavoidable, and remember that they are not permanent, this shifts your position, subsequent thinking and decisions. You may also have moved to the notion of an opportunity for learning. Resuming consistent practice as soon as possible, having self-soothed, is the key. When things have calmed, which they will, you can step back and look at the circumstances to decide the best way onwards. This is self-coaching.

Coaching requires presence. You know what it feels like when the person you are talking to is actually in the room, compared to being distracted! The practice of mindfulness helps us to be present more often in a time when there are many competing interests. For many people, it is a challenge to remain focused and concentrate. However, it is a skill that can be practiced resulting in improvements.

In being present, you can see things for what they are as you deepen your self-awareness with the circumstance of that moment. From this position, the best decisions can be made, resulting in the best outcomes. Remember that the best outcomes are not necessarily the ones you want (e.g. complete pain relief), but nonetheless are the only ones you could achieve at that time, considering the circumstances and the choices you had available to you. This highlights the importance of checking your expectations. If instead, you were to expect to do things the best way and to focus on then doing them in the best way you can, you are controlling the controllables. To focus on the end goal of complete relief means you are not actually putting your energy into the very action that could be helping. Do the basics well and the score takes care of itself.

Coaches are encouragers. They see people with strengths and potential to improve. They are also aware that you have weaknesses that need managing. But, we should mainly focus on strengths, because they deliver results and are more likely to bring you into a positive state—flow.

Spending more time in 'best states' shapes the types of changes that we want. Improving experiences are underpinned by neuroplastic changes in the neuroimmune and other body systems as we start to shift the predictions that these systems are making towards health over protection. Learning to encourage yourself can be a new skill for many people. Sometimes using phrases or mantras from others can help you. You may even hear it in their voice.

A simple practice that many people enjoy is to choose five trusted advisors. These can be people you know or know of. They can be alive or dead. This is your board. The people you turn to for advice if you have a question. It involves selection and then imagination. You imagine sitting around a table, or somewhere else you love to be, accompanied by your advisors. Then ask your question, and listen to what they say.

Building on what I said previously, coaching is communicating. You will increasingly notice what and how you say things to yourself and to others. In one way or another, we are all coaches: parents, teachers, managers, friends, therapists. At the heart of your coaching is your communication style. It is this style that determines your level of success.

In your journal, you can start taking note of the ways you notice you communicate with yourself and others. This may be uncomfortable, but an important way of developing yourself. You could ask others for feedback. This is common in different types of coaching: for example, sport, business. To appreciate the value of this type of exercise, you need to acknowledge the interrelatedness of life—we are all connected. The sense of who we are is built and maintained through others and interactions with others. This is one of the reasons why connecting or reconnecting with other people who matter to us is an important part of getting better.

Coaches are fastidious planners (see 'Planning, prioritising, and periodising'). They organise their time and help those they are coaching to organise theirs—bringing order and direction. To achieve your goals you need a plan. This is the way you get results, by having intent and following through on the necessary actions, rather than by accident. Each day, mapping out what you must do and the best times gives you a structure and makes it more likely you will act. You can also tick off each time chunk and feel a sense of satisfaction, building your inner motivation. This is self-encouragement, which you can add to with a kind word to self.

Coaching is an art and a science. There are important principles to follow, which I have outlined here, but you can do it in your own way. Self-coaching or working with your inner coach is no different from the way you would work with someone else. You are a person, to be heard, valued, encouraged, and guided to live a good life. To help a human being shape their life is also impacting on others they connect and come into contact with, having the inevitable ripple effect. This is powerful and takes it beyond the self, to something far greater than the self.

Encouragement points:

- Ultimately, you are your own coach.
- You are making decisions, and the quality of your decisions governs the quality of your life to an extent.
- There are consequences of each decision we make. Pluses and minuses.
- The more conscious we are of the consequences of our choices, the better informed we are to deal with what happens next.
- What kind of self-coach do you want to be?

Your approach

The way you go about understanding and overcoming your pain is individual. This is something you can control and decide. Practices, tools, and exercises are suggested, and you choose how you go about them.

You will already have some ideas. I will share some of mine for you to consider and perhaps build on your existing way, in your world. They tie closely with the principles in the preceding section (The Principles).

As ever, these suggestions come through a positive and strengths coaching lens. You could think of them as your self-coach. Whilst you can be supported, encouraged, and guided, ultimately it is your action that leads to results. Focusing on getting the best from the practices and reaching your potential by implementing them skilfully is self-coaching. My hope is that this book in its entirety will help you on this journey, as you build confidence and independence, underpinned by a belief in yourself.

Controlling the controllables

One way to make life smoother is to put your focus and energy into controlling the controllables. These are the things you can actually choose to influence.

They include your approach (hence this section), your attitude, your effort, your intent, and your style. You can decide all of these as you go about shaping a positive future. Of course, we have tendencies and ways of thinking already. Establishing whether they work or not is an important step. These have been conditioned as you have grown and developed, so there should not be any blame attached. However, on realising what works and what doesn't, you can focus on the former.

Things you cannot control are other people (they make their own decisions), the world and life that turns up the way it does regardless of your preferences. Trying to or even thinking that you can, takes you down a path of frustration and away from what you can control.

If you like, you can now make a commitment to your approach—a controllable one. Perhaps you have already done this. It can be useful to check in every once in a while to see that you are on track.

1. My attitude towards improving my health and life and easing my suffering is:
2. My style is:
3. My intent is:

Running your intent at the start of the day can help you set your course.

How will I approach the day?

In the morning it can be useful to set the tone with a few early wins and setting out your intent. What will be your style? This is your 'how'.

Some people like to start the day with a few movements: some breathing and a mantra. For example, I will do my best today, considering the circumstances. There are always circumstances, many of which are out of our control. Re-focusing on what you can do is important, as is accepting the reality of what is happening at that moment. This is not always easy, if ever. But you can certainly get better at doing it.

Another approach is to choose a strength to practice that day. Perhaps communication to self-compassion. Using the 1% rule can be helpful. This is when you aim to improve by 1%, which makes it manageable and achievable. Over a period of time, this accumulates to make a significant difference. This was the thinking of British cycling coach Dave Brailsford when he adhered to the principle of the aggregation of marginal gains.

Early wins in the day to feel some success come from acknowledging one or two activities that you have been able to achieve. You may not typically think of these as achievements (e.g. a shower, getting dressed, making the bed), but they are jobs done. In many cases, for the people I see, these are definite wins. Looking out for opportunities to succeed is inherent in getting better and overcoming pain. Then you can go a stage further and create these opportunities.

Coming through the predictive lens, by creating such an opportunity, you are forming a prediction error that you then seek to minimise by taking action. The feeling of success comes through this process, which you can build upon. The activity could be to walk a certain distance. You know you can do it within your window of tolerance, yet it will be a bit of a stretch. You give it your best by preparing in the right way (priming) and focusing. The main success comes from the planning and giving it a go. If you have done your best, you will get the outcome that is due from that effort (a controllable) plus the circumstances (an uncontrollable). Having this insight is key.

Little and often throughout the day

Just as you would eat several meals a day rather than eat them all in one go, practices are best used throughout the day. Many are skills that will improve over time and with repetition. The healthy skills are ones that you can choose to take forward, even as some of the more specific exercises can be left behind when you progress.

Some people like to do their exercises in one chunk. Perhaps even to get them out of the way! Great on doing them, but what about the habits and self-care for the rest of the day? There is still a need to practice consistently.

When you use the time chunking method with pauses between activities, you find that naturally you are practicing over the day.

Consistency

I use this word frequently. Being consistent builds momentum. Naturally, what you practice (your habits) consistently will bear fruit in one way or another. When you are clear on your picture of success and the steps to take each day, you understand the need for practice. It is important to you to feel and get better, making this a priority.

Sometimes we are blown off course or meet bumps in the road. This is inevitable. But with consistent practice, we are soon back on track.

A successful sports team will be consistent. You will hear the pundits talking about how they always do the basics well, and then add the pizzaz. The same applies to you and me in our day-to-day lives. If we focus on consistently doing the basics well, the results take care of themselves—Bill Walsh wrote a famous leadership book with such a title: *The Score Takes Care of Itself* (2009). This is the process over prize approach used by a number of top coaches whose insights have changed our understanding of achieving peak performance.

As an important aside, it is the thinkers Bill Walsh and Mike Pegg, already referenced, and others such as Steve Rollnick, Bill Miller, and David Cooperrider who can teach us not only great questions but how to ask them. The latter is key; a way of being in the moment of asking.

When you become distracted by thinking about your desired destination, you cannot see where to put your next step. It is understandable when you are suffering pain to want it to end. It is not your fault that this thought pops in over and over. But, it can take you away from the things you can do right now to be shaping that very positive future. This is very much part of the human condition—wanting to be somewhere else.

However, transforming suffering requires us to be present and face the challenges. There are strong messages in society about distracting from pain and suffering or trying to meet your needs with a quick fix of some kind. It's permissible to have a few drinks or a cigarette or something else. I am in no way criticising these ways of coping. There is no need for judgement here. Instead, I acknowledge that this is a way of you meeting your needs, which anyone else would use if they were in the same situation, me included.

There are many offerings for cures and quick fixes out there. If any of these worked well enough to be used across the globe to help the millions of people suffering, the scientists and clinicians in the pain field would know and be offering them. But as it stands, as much as you and anyone would like a rapid way of dealing with persistent pain, there isn't one. Instead, it is a journey forwards requiring consistent daily practice of healthy habits to create something better—a better life. This is no different from anything else that matters in life: relationships, work satisfaction, and fitness. All of these valuable parts of life require day-to-day practice and dedication.

To some people this may sound bleak. But, it is also a testament to our incredible human ability to learn and adapt to our circumstances, making changes in what we do to achieve results and live better lives.

Doing your best

I always come from the starting point that you, the person suffering persistent pain, are doing your best with the resources that you have. If this is not bringing the results that you want, then there is a need for more choices and ways to move forward. That is what should happen in your therapy sessions and from the many tools and practices in this book.

Doing your best is also a personal choice. Something you can control. You can decide each day that this will be your way.

Can over can't

Some people find that focusing on what they can do over what they can't is useful. It is certainly a feature of the work we do in the clinic. We look at what you can do and build on.

For example, you can walk for 15 minutes, but 20 minutes would result in too much pain. You know that the pain from walking 20 minutes is not due to any harm or injury, yet it is an experience where you have done worse than expected and hence not in line with your picture of success. To stay on track, you are trying to have good experiences. A good experience, which may feel better than expected at times, would be walking for 15 minutes, or even 10 minutes on some occasions. The key is that you have focused on what you can do, which can then be built upon in time as you progress forwards.

In another situation, you may want to go for a coffee with friends. You think that you won't be able to sit for the hour or so that you would all usually spend at the cafe. But you could sit for half an hour. This is a starting point, and viewing it as such is key. There is always a baseline where you begin and progress from. So, you decide to spend that half hour with friends, connecting and enjoying your coffee—this you can control. Then you decide to take your leave at the half-hour mark, whilst it is still a good experience, becoming a positive prior for the next time. On having a good time (not necessarily pain-free but on balance, positive), you will view the next occasion in a better light than if it were the other way around.

The whole experience of going out and socialising is a practice in itself. Opportunities to live life in the best way you can for that time, acknowledging the circumstances and being realistic, emerge in many ways. You could think about everything you do as a practice for improving your life, including how you look after yourself by taking the important rest and recharge breaks after each activity.

The process is dynamic, as is life. Things are always evolving and changing—impermanence. Each experience is new. You have never had this moment before. If you are feeling pain right now, you have never felt in the way that you are at this moment. And it will change. How can you bring this about?

What conditions can you create now? Like creating the conditions for a flower to grow.

Push or no push?

Many people tell me that they try to push through their pain. Sometimes this is because part of them believes that this is the way it should be done (social conditioning), perhaps they are in such need of making progress or simply because they want to be active. All are understandable, yet pushing often causes more pain.

The right message about pain and injury is that they have an unreliable relationship. Some take this as meaning it is ok to try and ignore the pain and push on through. There is a problem with this though. The more you do this, typically the more up and down the symptoms and suffering. Working within your window of tolerance is important.

To get better and ease pain, you need to create evidence that you are. In other words, have good experiences of being active and doing the things you want to. You curate and create these experiences—your practices, exercises, and daily activities. The way you do them in terms of the amount of time, when in the day, and how you recover afterwards are all important considerations.

The opposite also happens. Generally, good experiences can be built upon, so you have more good experiences. Painful experiences lead to more painful experiences. Why? Because each time we do something, how it is for us then becomes a past event playing a role in predicting the next one. Remember the predictive lens we are coming through.

You may like to review the pain section again at times as you progress through the book. This is something I encourage the people I work with to do, so as to deepen your practical knowledge of your pain. As you have different experiences and make your way onwards, more and more things fall into place.

By pushing I mean continuing to do something despite the pain, resulting in a sense of 'over-doing' it. This may mean it hurts more or you are exhausted and have to take action to recover. Essentially this would look like a very up and down pattern—over and under activity. Softening the curves makes a difference to your quality of life and how you keep motivated. It's a better ride.

For many people, there will be some pain. But on balance, you are able to consider what you have done as a positive and a success, take a break to adapt, and then continue with the next chunk of time (see 'Planning section'). I call this working within your window of tolerance, a term you will have read a few times earlier. You are working, training, living, and creating the conditions for a healthier self that includes lessening symptoms. Easing pain in a sustained way is always part of the programme. You can make this part of your approach.

The fact that you are doing something is a kind of push versus not doing it. But just not causing further suffering or the need to stop or avoid. Again, the positive or good experience is not necessarily pain-free, but it is a step in the right direction as on balance you are able to think about the activity as a positive.

Your window of tolerance will vary. This is why being flexible with your activity levels and consistent with rest and recovery time are both important. This is certainly true if energy is an issue for you—it is with many people who suffer persistent pain. Some people believe that they need to keep progressing and nudging along despite how they feel, because this is the goal that has been set. Usually this does not work out well, instead causing increasing pain and fatigue.

Being present, self-aware, and gaining insights into how you are in that moment allow you to check in and make your best decision. It may be that you need to walk a shorter distance that day, which is still a win for consistent walking. If your goals are dominated by distance or time only, then you may find yourself pushing when you actually need the opposite. The ability to gain insight and be present improves from mindful practice (see 'Mindfulness').

This is a common problem per se when people become focused on needing to cover a certain distance each week and force themselves regardless. There is a cost. The part of you that drives that behaviour is dominating the part of you that knows self-care must predominate for you to be successful in the long term.

When referring to pushing, I am also talking about how much strain you use with movements or stretches. Again, the way it feels will vary because each time you practice is a different moment. The dynamics of living mean that things are constantly changing, despite how they might appear to us or what we tell ourselves. This is why being present and checking in are so important before you start an exercise or an activity. Taking the moment to pause gives you the insight into how you are, which in turn leads to the best decision—What to do? How much to do? How to do it?

Stretching is a common exercise, despite the mixed findings in the research. Often this is due to different methodologies and groups of people who are being studied. So, how much should you stretch? Of course, the feeling of what it is like is only felt by you. I say to people that you can feel the stretch or the pull, but it should not be outside of your window of tolerance. You'll recall that your window will vary. Sometimes cues such as lengthening or feeling tension can help. Again, it should be experienced as something positive that you will repeat consistently. You may or may not be looking forward to the stretch, but you certainly do not want to be fearing it because of what happened before.

Curate good experiences that involve a challenge that you can overcome. There is often discomfort with this process as you gently bring flexibility back into your body systems as well as your tissues. But in doing this, you are aiming to bring flexibility back into your systems, shake beliefs that have become stuck with awareness, new thinking and actions and thereby making different predictions (updating them now that it is possible once again). You choose to act in and upon your world in a way that is meaningful, useful, and healthy and acknowledge what you are doing. That's the evidence.

Wisdom and making the best choices

You can argue that the quality of your day-to-day decisions determines the quality of your life. There are always consequences of every choice you make. Being aware of them by being present and making conscious decisions allows you to minimise surprise. There is always uncertainty of course.

Is this my best choice? Is this a wise choice? Both useful reflective questions you can use to self. The answer may not fit with your preferences, yet it does meet your needs. If you are aware of this, you can deal with the consequences. After all, if you jump in the river, will you complain that you are wet?

Making your best choice requires you to have a decent grip on reality: What is happening right now? How am I? What are my needs? What is it that I want to achieve? What is the next best decision?

Pausing to be present and aware then is a skill to practice. Being able to zoom in and then out means you can see the bigger picture. You can set a reminder to pause so that this becomes part of your way. You practice until it becomes a habit. Meditation helps develop this way of being.

Wisdom infers being closely in touch with the reality of the situation. For this, you must be present. Wisdom, presence, and awareness are entwined. There are specific examples. For instance, when you become aware that your self-critic is featuring in your inner world, you use wisdom to know that these are just thoughts. Further, you did not choose those thoughts or your mind. They are just happening and you are the one who is aware of the thoughts. You are not the thoughts.

Wisdom is not always popular. So, you will need courage to make wise decisions at times. Again, being aware of the consequences helps to choose.

Encouragement points:

- What are the things you can control?
- What is my intent?
- What will be my style? Approach?
- What is my philosophy?
- How can I do my best here, considering the circumstances?
- What can I do, and then build upon in line with my pictures of success and using my strengths?
- What is my next best decision, considering the circumstances?

Section 6 Practices and tools

Contents

Introduction

Welcome to the practices and tools section. As you will see, there are many. This is a selection of the ones I use more commonly with people I see. I have tried to recreate this via words, which I know has limitations, but I hope you can get a feel of how sessions would be for you. In one sense you are at an advantage because you can take the practices and start them immediately in your world.

Like any book or guide, this is a map. It is not the territory. The same is true of your experiences. They are the map not the territory. What do I mean by that? We have our own unique experience of ourselves and the world, not a direct experience of those things. Your perceptions at any given moment are a best guess about what is happening. Think about a map of your town. Then think about how a map of your town would have looked 100 years ago. The recent one will have been an updated version. We update our versions of ourselves and life in a similar way. But it is only ever a map. This truth offers possibilities. That is what you are now tapping into.

Coming to the clinic means together we practise and try things, but then you need to take them home. It is, of course, important that you feel the benefits and successes in your world, not just the clinic. This is the same for the online sessions that I do. As you can imagine, this way of working has become even more popular now with people across the globe connecting and working with me. However, I do love seeing people face to face.

With a book in your hand, it is down to you to do the work. That is when you will feel the benefit. The book is not the work. And, of course, it does nothing when sat on a bookshelf, even if it has been read. It is you who brings it alive in what you think and do, shining the light on where you are stuck, understanding that you can get unstuck and then going about it. Your new thinking and actions are what will make the difference.

'Overcoming pain is something you do …'

Within each section are the specified practices together with how to implement them, plus encouragement points at the end. My suggestion is that you earmark the ones that resonate and will fit with what you are doing. You may like to discuss them with your therapist or other people involved in your care so that it fits together.

The ones you are less sure about, you may like to give some of them a go anyway. There will be a reason why they don't seem as if they are for you, and this will be based on your existing beliefs. Your beliefs are just one version of events of course. Some will be helping you achieve the results you want and some will be limiting you. How can you discover which is which?

Firstly, be open to the fact that you can update your beliefs. Certain questions you can ask yourself will help: (1) What if I come from another perspective? (2) What would I suggest to a friend? (3) Is this really true? (4) What other possibilities exist? Being curious about the way you respond is part of getting to know yourself. Understanding the way your mind works is an essential part of achieving freedom from suffering. Then challenging your beliefs is important because some of those you hold could be taking you down the wrong path. The question is: am I getting the results that I want with my existing behaviours?

This is important for understanding and overcoming your pain, because it is your pain to understand and overcome. Whilst you are not your pain (you are the one feeling the pain), it is only you that lives and responds to the experience. No one else can feel your pain. It's yours to change by knowing why it is persisting and what in your life needs to change. This is empowering. It can also be challenging, but very possible.

It is important to point out that this does not and should not replace your existing therapy. I do not know your situation, and hence it should not be taken as direct advice. These are examples of ways that people have been able to ease their pain and suffering and live a better life in their own style. I am pleased to share them with you, but you should discuss what you are doing with your medical or healthcare practitioner.

Whichever you use and integrate into your life, I hope that they help you as they have helped others to move forward and shape a positive future.

Building your toolbox of practices and strategies gives you different options at different times. This is important as your needs will change as will circumstances. A practice that has worked before may not be so effective at another time. You need something else. Peak performers will toggle through their options until they find the one that is most suited. You can do the same.

Knowing the tools is one thing. Then you need the flexibility to use them, choosing the one you think will work best for you in a given situation and then switching if and when required. Your presence and self-awareness help you do this effectively. Further, you need the know-how. Just having a tool is no good without knowing the best way to use it.

For example, traditionally, people are given exercises to do. Perhaps they are drawn out on a piece of paper with some numbers. But how do you form the habit? When is the best time to do them? Should you always do those numbers or be flexible? How should you prepare? Recover? What if you don't complete them? And so on.

The know-how is key to success. I spend a lot of time with people on the know-how. The best way to use the tools and practices. So, I will share that here as well.

The principles

When it comes to the practices and tools, there are better ways of implementing and using them. I call this the know-how. It can make a significant difference to the outcomes. I describe to people how my wife could buy me an amazing drill and ask me to hang some pictures on the wall. Yet without the know-how, I still manage to make a mess of the job, even with the best drill in the world. I don't have the know-how (I really don't). But I could learn.

Not only is the way you implement your practices important but also your preparation. When there is a great deal of sensitivity and pain, the preparation and recovery time may be longer than the actual practice. Yet the ways you get ready are also key in feeling increasing control and getting better. You get yourself into a resourceful state rather than a fearful one. This is no different to an athlete or performer getting into a certain state to deliver their best. You can do the same.

In this section I outline some of the principles that we adhere to in the face-to-face sessions and programmes. They are based upon strengths-based coaching and the habits of peak performers.

Strengths-based coaching

I have been coaching for many years, starting as a cricket coach. Feedback from the kids I was working with (what they would say, how they would engage and improvements in performance of skills) and observing other coaches taught me a great deal. From what I saw, it was not simply a matter of time and repetition. There was a need for the right environment, quality feedback, encouragement, a willingness to learn, application, dedication, desire, intent, consistency, an openness to making mistakes, presence, and passion, to name a few.

I took this into my work as a registered nurse, where teaching patients was part of the day to day practice, including managing medication, medical devices and healthy skills. My subsequent degree in sport rehabilitation and sport science also included a significant amount of teaching and coaching

Some years later I was at a strengths-based coaching conference for people in human resources and organisational change. I like to spend time in other industries to understand their challenges in relation to health and well-being for performance. One talk stood out, and that was given by Mike Pegg, pioneer of strengths-based coaching in the UK. Afterwards I spoke to Mike, connected and ever since, he has played an enormous role in shaping my thinking and approach to helping people with persistent pain. Why?

For me, the treatment of pain was too focused on the pain. Sound silly? I had realised that much of how we feel and are is based upon what we are focusing on at that moment. Whatever fills your attention is your reality. Going back to my nursing years, my training emphasised helping people build their health rather than just preventing or treating a condition. The combination of these ideas and approaches made sense. What would happen if the person suffering pain focused on building health and wellness as a main thrust in getting better? The strengths-based coaching approach offered a method and a practical way of moving forward.

Strengths-based coaching is all about the person, you—the person first approach. As the coach or therapist, you see the person as autonomous, with a positive history, with strengths, past successes, and someone who is doing their best under particular circumstances. In Mike's words, we can help people to build on their strengths and achieve their picture of success.

Mike calls himself a positive encourager (https://www.thepositiveencourager .global/welcome-to-the-positive-way). I couldn't think of a better title. He talks about the positive approach to living life. This simply means the way we go about living would encompass a focus on what we can do, how we can contribute to others and the planet, and work towards a picture of success using our strengths whilst managing the consequences of our weaknesses.

With regards to persistent pain, I would rephrase this as: working towards your picture(s) of success using your strengths whilst managing the challenging moments in the best way you can. The notion of being positive is to try and keep your focus on what you want to achieve and the steps to take now in that direction. This could be any of the practices and tools in this book or those you already know and find helpful. Being positive is not saying that everything is great when it is not. It is about getting into resourceful states and finding a way.

Strengths-based coaching seeks to educate, encourage, and empower you to achieve success. You decide what that success looks like because this is about you building a better life, a good and fulfilling life with the support and guidance of a skilled therapist. The approach recognises that you are autonomous and competent, you will make choices and decisions, and that you can shape a positive future by creating the conditions at this moment. You take care of your future by taking care of now, the only moment.

Habits of peak performers

This is an area of intense interest and relevant to what you are doing. Typically, in healthcare, attention is upon the pathology, disease, or problem. Whilst we want to identify any of these for appropriate treatment, the vast majority of persistent pain cases exist without an obvious structural issue. The body tissues do not have the ability to produce pain. There will be a location in your body where you feel pain, but it is not actually coming from that place. Just as the film you watch in the cinema is not coming from the screen.

As you know now, persistent pain arises as a best guess by your body systems (nervous, immune, endocrine) essentially to maintain or re-establish homeostasis. All our experiences are being generated top-down. They are a version of events (your reality), not the event (the reality). You will recall the analogy of the map and the territory. We can take note of the map (experience or your reality) and then make the next best choice to update the map so that it better reflects the territory (the reality). This gives great hope because you are able to harness these systems to change your beliefs, thinking, and actions to change your perceptions. It seems that attention, for example, is a key player. This is something you can train with mindful practices.

You can choose to think about the types of practices people use to be successful and achieve consistent peak performance in their lives. This is not exclusively for elite athletes, professional performers, or CEOs of large companies. You and I can use these in our lives to achieve results. Such habits are littered through this book for you to use in your world.

Habits are the things you do each day, without much or any thought. They just happen. They also deliver certain outcomes down the line. How you are now is the result of the many habits you have: habits of thought and action. When you stop and review your situation, you gain insights into your current approach and the results. Having done this, you can establish what is working for you and what is not. This lines up with what matters to you. For example, if being healthy is important to you, your habits of eating well (most of the time) and exercising regularly are both contributing to the results that you want. I will address habits in more detail in the relevant section.

Being well is a way of being, a route of mastery. Daily practices that are consistently employed will bear fruit. There is no end point to such practices. Like cleaning your teeth—you would never stop, thinking that you have done enough now. This is a journey of living one's best life whatever the circumstances, keeping going just like an endurance event according to the standards you set yourself.

Circumstances

There are always circumstances. Some of these are out of our control, but must be considered whilst focusing on what you can control: attitude, effort, and intent. For instance, you could be doing your best in any given moment, but still be in pain or lose the game. Because the result was not the one you wanted, it does not mean that you have not done your best. Many people tell me that they must have done something wrong if their pain feels worse at any given moment (e.g. a flare up). Often this is not the case. There were just particular conditions meaning that pain was exactly what should have been felt. This can be hard to take on, especially if you have different beliefs. But when you can accept what happened, realise that nothing else could have happened under those circumstances, and then focus on this moment (that moment has gone), you will be free from the suffering caused by being tethered to the past.

The key is learning: what can you learn from that situation? And to move on because whatever happened is in the past. You cannot change it. So, let it go. This is a practice that you can learn. One of the major barriers to getting better is being caught up in the past or future, both of which obscure what is happening now. A peak performer represents the current situation in an empowering way and then focuses on the next best action. You can do the same.

Acknowledging what you can control and what you can't helps you to see the bigger picture. This is a skill in itself, being able to zoom out and see things for what they really are—all the contributing factors. Practicing meditation helps you to gain such insights and self-awareness. In noticing that you feel a particular way, or something happens, you are able to account for the main reasons why it was the way it was rather than another way. Then you can make your next best decision.

Your expectations also play a role (see Expectations). When they are out of sync with reality, you can feel bad as it seems things are not going your way. Again, if you can acknowledge the circumstances, you will be able to bring your expectations of yourself and the world in line with reality and resume your journey onwards towards something better.

Focus

You will have better outcomes if you are focusing on what you are doing. Thinking of the practices and exercises in the same way as learning can be useful. Being present and noticing what it is like gives you information about how well you are doing.

Focus is an important part of deliberate practice, a term used by Anders Ericsson and co-authors in their paper (1993) entitled, The Role of Deliberate Practice in the Acquisition of Expert Performance. Ericsson was a Swedish psychologist who studied human expertise and performance.

His work was misquoted, resulting in the belief that 10,000 hours of practice would result in him becoming an expert. What he was actually saying was that the quality of practice mattered. A more recent paper discussed the findings over the years and made recommendations for the future (2019) with regard to the most effective forms of training.

This is the point I am making here. For your best outcomes, you need to be engaged with what you are doing. Turning towards your body and how it feels as you move takes courage but is essential in transforming your experience. You come to realise that your experiences are essentially what you are attending to, and you become more skilful at where you put your attention. Like a spotlight. This needs to be within your window of tolerance, which will grow.

Some people find it hard to focus. Your mind wanders off. Mindful practice helps to become better at realising when this happens, so you can bring your mind back to what you are doing. Paying attention is a skill of being well with people reporting a greater sense of happiness when they can pay attention (Killingsworth & Gilbert, 2010). You are also more likely to do a better job, bringing your own level of satisfaction. You can certainly be pleased with your efforts once you have completed a practice in line with your picture of success.

If you tend to be distracted easily, you may decide to set up the environment in your favour. Turning off devices, for example, or going into a room where it is easier to focus on what you are doing. Practicing meditation, you will probably want to be somewhere quiet, perhaps warm, but not so comfortable that you nod off! You may need sleep, but you are not practising.

Ericsson's work could be seen as practice for experts (musicians), but I would argue that we can all use the habits of peak performers and experts to better our lives. You can set your intent to practise in the best way you can, considering the circumstances. The key principles that he laid out were: (1) individualised training for an individual by a trained teacher (2) the goal(s) are communicated by the teacher and the trainee can represent this internally whilst training (3) the teacher describes the practice for that particular goal, which gives the trainee immediate feedback when they try (Ericsson & Harwell, 2019).

In the therapeutic setting and at home, you can apply the same principles. You have an individualised programme of practices, exercises, and tools that have been tailored to meet your needs and are the steps towards achieving your goals. These goals are chosen by you, which is one point of difference. They are chosen because they have meaning and are important to you—value-based. You know what you want to achieve and have some sense of it. Finally, as you practise and are present, you know what you are trying to do and by paying attention can realise when you are doing well and not so well. In the latter case, you can then make corrections accordingly. There is always something to learn.

'But here's the lesson I learned.' Bill Walsh (2009)

Life is a winding road

Life is full of ups and downs. Overcoming pain is no different. There is no straight path to a better and healthier life. It is a route full of obstacles that can become opportunities—this is a way of representing them that is empowering. Once you can accept this is the way, you can put your energy into the skills and practices that deliver results. This is the importance of daily habits that accumulate and yield positive changes in time.

For example, doing an exercise one day will not create any visible changes or make the movement much easier the next day. Or the next. But if you were to practice every day for a few months, then you will start to feel the difference. It can take around three months for any significant change. Life is cumulative and the direction depends on the daily choices you make.

So how can you keep going when there is no obvious and immediate reward? And in a world where instant gratification and quick fixes are promised. When it comes to health and wellness, there are no quick fixes! Just repetition. It just has to be important enough to be a priority. When you have a really good reason, you will find a way—the importance of meaning.

Some find this challenge appealing and some don't. It's a preference that has developed. However, accepting that this is how it works means you can get into the business of taking those first steps. How you think about your pain (and everything else) is largely determined by the society and culture in which you are embedded and what you have learned and been conditioned to think. This is the same for everyone. But are your thoughts in line with what we know about pain (the reality versus your reality) helpful?

The Stoics have much to say on this matter, as do other philosophical schools of thought such as Buddhism. I am not a Buddhist, but the tenets, insights, and practices offer ways of dealing with life in a compassionate way to benefit all. They all agree on the fact that life is full of suffering and there are ways of easing suffering. This starts with the way we think, which is based on our beliefs. Our beliefs stem from what we have been conditioned to think and understand about ourselves and the world, together with past experiences.

Some cultures view pain as part of life, even to be embraced as an experience. In the West, we try to avoid pain, living the most comfortable lives that we can. However, with the inevitability of pain and suffering, without tools to deal with them, and with the expectation that we should not feel pain, the suffering grows. This was illustrated in Dr Paul Brand's book, The Gift of Pain, which tells his story of working with people who had leprosy.

Long thought that the sores and disfigurement were due to leprosy, Brand realised that the injuries, subsequent infections, and often early deaths were caused by people's inability to feel pain. Essentially, pain being protective means that there are healthy boundaries in which we remain so that body integrity is maintained. Without pain, there is no safety net, resulting in a high risk of injury and the subsequent effects.

A small stone in your shoe unfelt could damage the skin of your foot. Without realising, this cut can become infected and inflamed. Undetected, the infection persists and affects the whole foot, and so on. If you don't feel pain, you cannot know that something needs addressing or protection for healing.

At the other end of the spectrum is persistent pain, the focus of this book. You could argue that whilst someone experiencing no pain is always in potential danger, another person with ongoing pain feels danger when there is none in most cases.

Overcoming pain is a winding road. It continues to wind in different ways—different challenges. But, when you have travelled the twists and turns, learning all the way and becoming more skilful through practice, when you encounter future challenges, you are prepared. The impact is less. Once you have had a pain, you may feel it in a similar way (it cannot be the same) in times to come, but not necessarily because anything 'bad' has happened. Instead, there are some circumstances like a time before that are sufficient for the prediction of pain as the best explanation for what is happening now.

The goal is to move forward in a positive way. To improve your life, knowing that there will be ups and downs. But, now you have skills and know-how to deal with them and move on, tied closely with the insight of impermanence (see below). This gives you the confidence to make decisions and go about living your best way. In all cases, it is possible to make life better. In some cases the pain resolves.

Window of tolerance

Working within your window of tolerance means that you are having good and better experiences to build upon. What does this mean? By curating your actions, you are setting yourself up to achieve a win. This ties closely with bringing your expectations of what you can do in line with reality, which is key for success moving forward (see Expectations).

The window of tolerance is when you are active at a level that means the quality of what you are doing is high, you can focus and the symptoms (pain) are not interfering. It also means that when you are finished, you can continue with your daily plan.

To do this well requires presence and acknowledgment of the circumstances of the moment. There can be a strong part of you that says you should be doing more or is critical of the way you are acting. Another part knows that to be successful, you need to do the basics well and stick to the plan. This is the caring and wise part of you.

Your window will vary from moment to moment. There are many variables, most of which we don't have conscious access to. All we have is the quality of what it is like right now. There is no read out from the body. This is why being present and checking in with curiosity is important, so you can make your best decision whilst focusing on process over prize (see section: Process over prize).

Keeping within the window, and then exploring the edges at the right times (when you are feeling safe and have consistently practised, building a positive history) means your activity levels will grow organically without any forcing or pushing. These do not typically work well, instead causing flare ups and making the journey very bumpy.

Graded exercise that is rigid causes problems. This approach does not acknowledge changing circumstances and hidden variables. Used for ME and chronic fatigue syndrome (CFS), this was an approach that brought about much suffering despite what people were feeding back. Similarly with persistent pain, pushing through does not work. Instead, you must work with yourself and your body (they are one of course), not against it, dancing rather than fighting.

Step by step

The step to focus on is this one. There is only this one, right now. If you become lost in the future, you cannot take care of this moment, the real moment. Same with the past. Both are stories we can become lost in and influenced by.

To create a better future, you must make your best decision now. Step by step.

Having a plan makes this possible, plus knowing how to create a habit. Both are fully addressed in the relevant sections.

I was running down a steep hill on a rocky path. A gate was in the distance. That was where I was heading. That was my short-term goal. To get there, I needed to focus on where my next step would be, scanning the ground ahead. If I was to look too far and concentrate on the gate, the risk of tripping and falling was great. This is an analogy for the need to focus on this moment, this step. Then the goal takes care of itself.

Impermanence

In the Impermanence section, you will find a more in-depth look at this Buddhist principle that explains how life is possible.

Beyond this, I wanted to mention an important point. When I ask people about treatments they have had or techniques they have tried, sometimes they tell me that they worked but only for a short period of time. When you consider the truth of impermanence (things are always changing no matter how it may seem), you will understand why anything that is done will have a short-term effect.

Of course, the overall aim is to have a better life, as defined by you. However, there will always be ups and downs, and there will always be suffering in life. But you can also ease your own suffering by understanding yourself more deeply.

If you take a pill, you may have relief for a time. If you have an injection, you may have relief for a time. If you have some kind of hands-on treatment, you may have relief for a time. And so on. No matter the relief, there will be another bump in the road down the line. This is normal. When you can accept this truth and focus on ways to live well, build health, and deal with the difficulties more and more skilfully, life gets better. You drop the resistance.

No quick fix—no fix at all

Nowadays we can order stuff and it arrives quickly. Same day if you choose. I can download my favourite movie or album. Food will be delivered within the hour. Now, now, now—I can't wait. This is a strong message from society, and it can be useful. But not always.

If you expect your health or feeling better to be as quick, you will always be disappointed. Again, it is a matter of expectation and reality mismatch. How many problems does this cause in life?

There are no quick fixes for persistent pain, as much as we would love there to be. There are no hacks, despite what is promised. Getting better and overcoming pain is an active process, sometimes helped by passive treatments, of understanding, learning, and creating new habits. It takes time, perseverance, and courage. It is difficult and fraught with challenges. But with the right support, encouragement, and guidance, it is very possible.

Going a step further, I believe that there is nothing to fix. You certainly don't need fixing. Common parlance talks of fixing, like you are a car or something else that is broken. The problem with this language is that we shape our experiences with the words we use. Therefore, it becomes a strong message to self about your perceived state: I am broken and need fixing. This puts the onus on someone else doing the work for you, which creates an expectation-reality mismatch.

Instead, my suggestion is to use language that focuses on what you are doing to shape a positive future, full of encouragement. In other words, instead of fixing, you learn to create the conditions by making smart choices consistently. From these conditions emerge the kinds of results you desire. They cannot be willed any more than a flower can be willed by looking at a seed. You plant the seed, nourish it, and allow the growth.

Encouragement points

1. There are principles to follow that will help you use the tools and practices in the most skilful way.
2. The principles are the know-how, or ways to best implement your programme.
3. It can be useful to refer back to these principles once you have designed your programme and made your plan.

Process over prize

'Focus on what you can control, the process, and not what you can't, the prize. Do the former as well as you can, and the latter takes care of itself.' RS

Great teams and performers consistently do the basics well. They focus on their strengths and manage the consequences of their weaknesses (Pegg, 2012). You will see this in sporting tournaments that span across a season. As the season nears its climax, the teams and players who were consistently doing well sometimes falter as they succumb to the pressure. The basics seem to go out of the window. What is happening?

The players lose focus and start to be influenced or pressured by the prize rather than continuing to do what has been working. In one sense it is a distraction. The manager then tries to get them to refocus on the process over the prize, which takes care of itself when the former is done well.

The same principles apply to us on a day-to-day basis. We keep thinking about what we want, the end goal, rather than the necessary steps to take right now. As human beings we have this tendency, but undoubtedly we can train ourselves to refocus on what we must do now in order to bring success. To be able to pay attention is a skill that we can improve. One of the best ways is to practise daily and moment-to-moment mindfulness, which some now refer to as focused attention training. Interestingly and relevant is the fact that paying attention is a skill of being well. The more we are able to pay attention, the happier we report being according to a study entitled: A wandering mind is an unhappy mind (Killingsworth & Gilbert, 2010).

In a society that values the prize above all else and encourages competition over collaboration, it is natural to gravitate towards thinking about the result. Schools talk of values and developing the person, yet publish their results as the main indicator of success. However, the grades don't reveal the suffering caused by anxiety and pain that are the price. They are the ones I see. From the outset, this is how youngsters are being trained to think, taking these beliefs into adulthood, their work, and health. The energy and expectations are in the wrong place and need to be unpicked.

Working environments that are competitive over all else create huge amounts of stress. Bonus-driven roles can require one person to beat another. Some may feel that they thrive in such an environment. But if there can only be one winner, what about all the rest? What is the cost of there being one winner? Values are put aside in order to win. What is the effect of this on people, even the winners?

This is not to say that competition per se is bad. There just needs to be perspective taken (the bigger picture) and success be measured using different parameters: for example, effort, attitude, approach, as well as a placing. There is also a need for fulfilment. Are you pursuing your purpose? Feeling fulfilled in what you are doing is very healthy. Many people consider themselves successful because of their wage packet or the car they drive, yet deep down they are unhappy. I have seen many such people who have lost their way.

The constant comparison that has become permissive and the norm is causing immeasurable harm. People feel that they are not good enough, not worthy of happiness and joy, and sometimes deserving of pain and suffering. What kinds of messages are these? We must change the narrative in our society. The stress is damaging at all levels, largely because of its frequency and intensity. How about messages such as: you are perfect as you are, you could not be any other way, you are good enough, you are doing your best.

A different narrative that you can use:

The only step I can take towards my picture of success is this one, right now. What is the best step I can take at this moment? In doing this repeatedly, I am now creating the conditions for a positive future. I cannot make that better future manifest by simply thinking about it or dreaming of that imagined future. It gives me direction, but I am not there yet—yet being the key word.

You can choose to focus on what you can control rather than what you cannot. You can control your approach, set your expectations, choose your attitude and intent, and the action that you take. You cannot control the future because it does not exist except in your mind as a guide or practical plan (what you want to achieve and what you don't). You also cannot control the world or other people. People who try to control these are perpetually frustrated and create a huge amount of stress for themselves. They can also feel like they are continually failing as they are unable to achieve the things that they want to (see Setting expectations).

Deciding to focus on the process means that you gather wins along the way that further motivate you to continue on that path. You can acknowledge and affirm your efforts and always consider the surrounding circumstances. For instance, on a given day you may be more tired. As a result, you decide to change your plan, reduce the number of reps, and increase the recharge time. You could be frustrated that you have had to make these changes, or you can accept the circumstances and be mindful of making sensible adjustments. You are doing your best in the light of this and keeping my direction. To force through is more likely to cause you to go off course.

As I have said on many occasions, consistency is key. The levels of practice may vary, but overall are on an increasing trend. For this to happen, you must be consistent with your planning and actions, each day, every day, building onwards.

Encouragement points

- It is important to know where you want to go—your goal or picture of success.
- But then focus on the best step now, at this moment.
- When you put your energy and intent into doing the basics consistently well, the prize takes care of itself. Just like a successful sports team.
- You want to get to the top of the mountain. But don't forget that there is a mountain.
- It is this step now that matters.

Sessions and who you work with

'Chronic pain is a specialist field. Make sure you find someone with the right background, approach, skills and knowledge.' RS

There comes a point when you may need help. You decide to go and see someone. But who? And why? You will have your reasons, which you hope to share at the first meeting. Then you get on with the treatment programme that has been presented as a way forward, working towards your goals. This is a very broad description and the way therapy unfolds varies enormously depending on the type of therapist you are working with and their approach. In reality, the basis of the therapy sits within the relationship between the two people, their beliefs, and how they come together. It is a dynamic.

It is worthwhile thinking about your sessions, primarily so that you get the most out of them, translating into positive action in your world—what happens in the clinic room is in a bubble. This is one of the benefits of online sessions. You are already in your environment, which is playing a role in your pain experience. By taking action immediately, you are able to start creating the conditions for a positive future.

Who to see

The people you may go to see could be your doctor, a physiotherapist, a massage therapist, an osteopath, a psychologist, a therapist, or someone else. It depends on who you think will help.

Who do you think can help you?

Some people seek help because they are persuaded to do so. A partner may encourage, request, or even 'order' an appointment. They may even book it for you. For things to start in the best way though, it is you who must want to get an opinion and be open to ideas about what can help you. It is you who must come to the realisation that what you are doing right now is not delivering the results you want.

Who is the best person to see for persistent pain? It is someone who is professionally trained and understands persistent pain.

This sounds obvious I know. But there is a huge mismatch between the number of therapists treating chronic pain and the number of therapists who truly understand chronic pain. Put another way, would you go and see a clinician about your heart disease who does not specialise or have knowledge and understanding of it?

Pain is a speciality, especially chronic pain. The term pain specialist means that the professional has specific knowledge and skills to help you understand and overcome your pain.

Consider how much thinking and checking goes into buying a car, a pair of running shoes, a phone, or whatever you are into. Then, how much goes into thinking about who to best see for your health? Hopefully more!

It is easy to read people's profiles online in most cases. You can see whether they specialise in pain. Their background and training are sometimes stated, and of course you can ask. Once you have identified the person who you think is right for you, the next step is booking an appointment.

People you might see

There are many different therapists and clinicians you may have seen. In the ideal world, they would be saying the same things to you, giving you hope and encouragement. They would also be using the same model of pain to be consistent. Unfortunately, this is not what happens.

Each practitioner will have their own experiences and knowledge base, but essentially will want to help you move forward and relieve your symptoms.

There is no absolute healthcare professional for persistent pain, which is part of the problem. The ideal person has training and experience in a range of relevant fields, built on a foundation of understanding pain. They will also have a way of being and an approach that resonates with you. You are made to feel like the centre of their world, heard and seen. They listen to you and help you understand both your experiences and any objective findings, drawing the two together. This is an art form based on a trusting relationship. There is a togetherness that is important, walking a path together.

I often think about the characteristics that make a Pain Coach. You know about Pain Coaching now from the previous section. Commonly they include compassion, empathy, patience, wisdom, kindness, practical, self-awareness, and calmness. They have a deep knowledge of pain and human behaviour, plus a large toolbox of practices, exercises, strategies, and techniques to offer you. Importantly, they have the ability to show you how to best implement the tools in your world. It is not enough to just give someone exercises to do or tools to use. You need the know-how to get the best results.

People do wonder who is best to go and see for help. That there is no one profession that can make this confusing. My suggestion is to take on board the comments above, plus discover if the potential therapist or clinician understands the latest thinking in pain. Do they know about and use the contemporary model? Are they focusing on you? Is it a truly holistic approach?

Who are the professional helpers? Remember that they should be specialists in pain to help and guide you. Further, they need to be able to apply the modern knowledge about pain in a practical way for you, so that you have a full understanding and the know-how. A clinician may have a great appreciation of pain science, but this is only helpful if it can be applied and practised. It's from the actions that results arise. Here are some of the common professions:

- Your doctor (or GP): initial appointment, organising appointment referrals, managing medication and other kinds of support.
- A pain doctor (consultant): specialise in diagnosing conditions and administering medication and interventions to help relieve pain.
- Specialist pain physiotherapist: help you understand your pain, ease your symptoms and then move on to shape a positive future in practical ways.

- Pain Coach (PC): this is the concept I have been developing over the past 15 years or so. It is the essence of this book, although primarily a way of being with people who are suffering persistent pain. The PC sees your strengths and potential to shape a positive future by helping you understand your pain and then guiding and encouraging you in practical ways to achieve success.
- Psychologist: to help you with your thoughts and feelings about your pain.
- Therapist: there are many forms of therapy (hundreds!), which can make the choice overwhelming. Perhaps it is a combination of the person and their approach. This means taking the plunge (using your courage) and seeing if it feels right. Is the therapy meeting your needs? Does it feel right?

The person or people you work with will depend on your needs.

A note on trauma

How much is trauma at play with your chronic pain?

There has been a huge amount of work looking at trauma and its effects. Some people believe this is at the heart of chronic health problems, which can be true but it is not definitive. A blanket belief that prior trauma, particularly adverse childhood experiences (ACEs), will cause issues later in life would not account for the fact that some people develop resilience as a matter of the events and how they coped (Bonanno, 2021).

All prior experiences shape who and how you are now. Understanding this and your past can be helpful to see this and to decide what is working for you and what is not. This is where a therapist can be helpful, although some people discover it themselves or through conversations with other clinicians, friends, or even strangers.

There is no one way, which is why listening to your unique story is the key start point.

In your story perhaps there are ACEs or maybe the pain began following a traumatic episode:

- accident
- injury
- loss (e.g. death of a loved one, made redundant)

- illness (e.g. covid)
- stress (e.g. bullying at work, overloaded with life's demands, an onerous self-critic)

There is trauma with a big T (huge, so-called life-changing events, and trauma with a little t (day-to-day situations and events, sometimes in the wake of the big Ts). Trauma can also follow trauma. Following one significant event, there can be a sequence of situations and episodes that are further traumas. For example, treatments that do not bring about the desired effect, feeling disbelieved, reminders of the inciting event, and nightmares.

As the time of suffering continues without direction (towards something better), there can be an increasing number of triggers or cues associated with the pain. Whilst similar patterns and habits are in play, this continues, which is why understanding and then creating new patterns forges a positive way forward.

One consequence of trauma is post-traumatic stress disorder (PTSD). Symptoms of PTSD include:

- flashbacks; it feels like it is happening again
- intrusive thoughts
- nightmares (vivid, strange, scary, terrifying)
- pain, nausea, sweating
- overwhelming emotions
- easily upset, irritated
- feeling panicked
- aggression
- disturbed sleep

There are other experiences, but these are common—not necessarily all of them. If you think you are experiencing PTSD, I would strongly advise you to seek help as this will hold up your healing and recovery.

When I first meet someone, I am alert to these experiences so I can suggest appropriate help as soon as possible.

The first appointment

I tend to call these sessions or meetings, preferring to move away from medicalisation. Why? Because your route forward is towards health, wellness, and a better life that is away from the medical world. You focus on what you want rather than what you don't.

I also consider the first meeting to be a friendly conversation with illuminating points (thanks to Mark Epstein's client for this one), when I am mainly listening. This is your opportunity to tell your story, in your own words and in your own way. My role is to create a safe environment where you feel that you can speak freely. This is your session about you.

A good therapist will give you time and space to describe your experiences but also ask you to share your concerns and worries. These can then be addressed directly, there and then.

Here are some things you may like to know:

1. Why is my pain persisting?
2. What can I do?
3. What can you do to help me?
4. Is there a time line we can follow?

In the initial session, I aim to gain insights into you and your experiences, and to understand your concerns and know the kinds of things you want to achieve—your picture of success. I will then start to help you understand your pain and symptoms. It must make sense and have meaning for you. Finally, I will outline a way forward, describing the programme.

There is an examination of the way you move and enact your pain following this conversation. By observing the way you move, testing muscles, sensation, and body sense, I can see how you have adapted—a snapshot. These are patterns that are not separate from the way you think and perceive. You think with your body and according to your biological state, explaining why limited or painful movement and pain itself can have such an impact on the sense of who you are and how you feel.

We are seeking to understand your lived experience: what it is like being you. With persistent pain, life is more difficult. Instead of a transparent body that you can rely on and trust without thought, it becomes a source of anxiety, pain, and misery. You may be thinking about how or if you can do certain things that beforehand you would have done habitually, without thought.

Now you want something different and better.

The stepping stones to the next sessions and the onward journey include trust in the clinician/therapist, feeling that you have been validated and heard, and seeing a way forward. You have clarified what you want to achieve (your vision), why it matters (purpose and values), your strengths, and now you move on to the 'how' as you collaborate with your healthcare professional.

Follow-up sessions

The follow-up sessions bring the content and the practices to life as you start working towards your picture of success. Your clinician or therapist will have ideas to share with you and you may have some particular areas you want to work on. Coming through a coaching lens, I will ask you what has been going well so we can study your successful styles and then find out about the challenges you have been facing. An important rule of thumb is that wherever and whenever you feel irritated, anxious, angry, frustrated, or pain, it reveals the work to be done.

Other appointments

You may be having other appointments for investigations, check-ups with doctors, and attending other therapies (e.g. treatment for PTSD, depression, or something else). You may have been on, or are waiting for a pain management programme, where you have access to a range of clinicians and therapists in one place—the multidisciplinary team or MDT.

The key is for all the members of the team to be communicating well. It can be confusing when therapists and clinicians are giving different messages. Naturally, this can happen because people use different models and have different beliefs. If there are conflicting messages, you can ask for clarification. The most important thing is for you to feel that you are at the centre of the programme and empowered to take the actions needed to overcome your pain.

Too many therapists spoil the broth

Persistent pain throws up many anxieties about the future. The world and the opportunities within the world appear differently; often narrowed or threatening. This can create a feeling of vulnerability. Consequently, some people find themselves visiting many different kinds of therapists and doctors, seeking answers or perhaps a cure. Often, we look for the types of answers that confirm our beliefs, dismissing those that don't even though they may be right. This poses a problem as we can find ourselves going down the wrong path.

How do you know what is right for you? This is a personal question as each person has their own path determined by their particular needs. When you have clarified what you want to achieve, the needs you must meet and the conditions to create, you can decide who you must work with in order to be successful.

An important question to yourself is, am I getting the results that I want? Part of this is to know whether your expectations are realistic or not. You may need to discover this by having a conversation about change, which would typically be part of the coaching process.

If you are getting the results you want, meaning that you are heading in the right direction, your focus will be on maintaining momentum and direction. If not, you may want to consider alternative actions and then re-measure your outcomes within a realistic time frame.

Encouragement points

- Work with a therapist or clinician who understands persistent pain—it is a specialist area.
- You may need to work with several different therapists to have your needs met, depending on your situation.
- If the messages from therapists become confusing or conflicting, ask for clarification. You may need to reduce input from some.
- This is your journey and you should feel like you are in the driving seat.
- Sessions are yours and must be meaningful and useful as you work towards your picture of success. They are signposts as you do your work in your world to improve your life.

Planning, prioritising and periodising

'Having a plan can make the difference between taking positive action and not.' RS

To be successful, you need a daily plan to follow. You also need a structure for the day. This way you can do all the things you want and need to, plus have the necessary breaks to manage your energy. All actions are geared towards your picture of success, and you can see this when you look at your plan. Some people like to colour code their plan, which gives an overview of the balance of activities. Too much of one colour may need addressing.

How do you do this? I suggest drawing upon the habits of peak performers. What does an athlete do to achieve the best performance? If you look at an athlete's schedule, you will see it is highly organised. They can tick off each activity and feel a sense of success and pride. You can do the same, acknowledging your efforts—process over prize.

The approach you take is tied closely to the plan you follow. There needs to be some flexibility. Unexpected things come up and need your attention, meaning you may have to juggle. If you are too rigid on having to do certain practices or exercises, and then you are unable to for some reason, you need to be able to cope and resume practise when you can. There are times when rest and recovery need priority, or a modification of the amount, or intensity (dosing). As you become a skilled self-coach, building self-awareness and listening to your needs, you will make better decisions. Even if they are not the ones you would usually make.

When you focus on the process over the prize, being able to roll with changes becomes easier: what is your best decision right now, considering the situation you are in? You know that you are doing your best, given the circumstances, but sometimes you have to deviate from the plan. Accepting this is important—these are the circumstances. You may be frustrated or concerned that you haven't practised, but knowing that this is fine and that you'll be able to pick up again soon makes you feel better. You may even learn something by changing the routine. You will definitely learn something if your approach is one of curiosity and compassion.

Planning

Make a list of all the things you need and want to do. For instance, a morning routine to get the day going in a positive direction, particular movements or exercises, household chores, attending to the kids' needs, working, meeting friends, and sending emails. You can keep a log of all the things you do each day to see how much you actually achieve and note what you get up to. It's an interesting experiment that I would recommend you only do for one day.

Having a plan makes it much more likely that you will follow through and take action. You can also share your plan with others so that they know when you are available. This can be especially useful in the workplace or when you are working from home and others can access your diary. Sticking your coloured plan to the fridge tells your family or housemates what you are doing and when—as long as you want them to know!

Prioritising

Once you have your list of things to do, you can prioritise. A simple way to do this is using A, B, C … 1, 2, 3 as recommended by Alan Lakein, the time management author. Time is our most valuable and finite resource.

Take your list and categorise each task as an A, B or C: A = very important, must be done, B = somewhat important, needs to be done soon, C = not very important, can wait. Each day you can re-categorise as you need to because things do change.

Next, look down your As and number the 1, 2, 3, 4, and so on. Then do the same for your Bs and Cs.

Now you have your prioritised list of things to do that can be fitted into your schedule.

The time slot lengths will vary depending on your situation and the task. As a guide, peak performers will work or practise for 45 to 90 minutes and then rest for 10 to 15 minutes (Stulberg & Magness, 2017). They will repeat this throughout the day, having a longer break in the middle for lunch.

Working out how long you can do something is an important practice. This is commonly known as Pacing, so I will use this term (see Pacing section).

Periodising

You may decide to start the day in a particular way (see Morning routine) because this gets you into the right mindset and deals with common experiences such as stiffness and grogginess. Then you set your lunch break and dinner time. This gives you a basic structure to fit in time slots on either side for the different activities and tasks. These are your periods of activity with recharge and rest breaks punctuating your day (see Energy). Now that you have planned and prioritised, you can periodise, or chunk.

Chunking your time is a phrase I often use with the people I am working with. We can focus on the current chunk and what we are doing in that time rather than the overwhelming prospect of a whole day. This makes it feel more achievable and we can tick it off afterwards. A win that you can acknowledge and log! And then onto the next.

Sticking to your plan and being consistent are both important. Remember that this is a way of dealing with the ups and downs and uncertainties. By doing things well now, you are taking care of your future and you will be able to progress.

There are times when you feel better and will be tempted to do more. This is when we need to remind ourselves to be disciplined and maintain course, continuing to create good experiences to build upon. Focus on what you need rather than what you want—what is my best decision now? And now?

Planning new activities

When opportunities arise, normally you would want to take them. For instance, to go out with friends, play with the kids, do some gardening, or go for a run. However, in a chronic pain state, you can find that you have shifted into an energy-saving mode, which is felt as a loss of motivation and a lack of energy. Your brain does this for you, shifting your body systems into a saving mode, cutting back on things that use energy.

The two most expensive activities in terms of energy are moving and learning. This means you may not feel like doing anything or seeing anyone, even though moving and connecting with people will often make you feel better. So, when you want to explore and be more active, this is a positive. You just need to do it in the right way to make it a good experience that you can build upon.

Using the 'can over can't' principle (see Your approach), you think about what you can do, considering your current tolerance and ability level. I will use an example to illustrate.

Friends ask you to go for a coffee at the local cafe. You want to go and are excited about catching up. Then you worry about how to get there and how you will sit with them in those uncomfortable chairs. What to do? You could say no, again. Or you could work out a way of being successful and view this as an opportunity to take a step forward. You will need to accept that to do this, it will need to be in a particular way, but if you do it well, then you will be able to build on this next time, working towards your picture of success.

This is an opportunity to practice. In fact, everything you do is practice for the next time. Life is cumulative and continuous. What you do now shapes what will come. Taking care of this moment takes care of the next one.

How will you get there? It is a short drive, but this would cause you a fair amount of pain (in your thinking because of prior experiences), making the sitting harder. You have an idea. You will ask your friend to pick you up. That deals with that issue and the pressure of driving and trying to find a space (it's always busy around there). You decide to work on increasing your driving distances on another day.

You can sit for 20 minutes and that is fine. You need to move at that point, and if you do, you can usually sit for another 15 to 20 minutes. Let's say 15 minutes—underplay rather than overdo so that you are curating your own successful practices. So, that is about 30 to 35 minutes you can be in the coffee shop. Then you will need to leave and get a lift home.

If you talk to your friend and explain what you can do and how they can help, that will set everyone's expectations and you have a plan that you can fulfil—minimising uncertainty and hence feel more secure in what you are doing.

You will have your own examples of situations, resources that you have, and ways that others can help (see Family and friends). It may be useful to create a few plans for things you can do, which you will build upon in time by following these principles. And remember, once you have made your plan, stick to it, let go of the temptation to stay longer, finish in the mindset of stopping one rep short (and wanting more), and acknowledge your success. You are creating your own positive history to draw upon next time.

Making adjustments—being flexible

It is inevitable that you have to change your plans or tweak what you are doing. Whilst this can cause some frustration or self-criticism, being flexible is an important skill. There are two things to remember: (1) you are doing your best (2) the way forward is not a straight line.

Doing your best does not mean always pushing or following the plan to the letter. In fact, pushing is rarely a fruitful approach as it can have a cost. Your best means the right attitude, approach, and mindset as you put your energy into the most profitable places more often than not, keeping your picture of success in mind and focusing on what needs to be done right now. This is something you can control.

The concept of good enough introduced by Winnicott, a paediatrician and psychotherapist, can be helpful. This takes unnecessary pressure off as you strive to do your best and focus on what you can control rather than what you can't.

Practicing self-compassion (see Compassion) is an important part of over-coming pain. If and when the critical voice appears—that part of you that is usually harsh, unkind, unsupportive—you can increasingly recognise that voice and realise that it is just one part of you, and that there are many other parts that are caring, encouraging, and motivating. More on the practical elements later.

Recovery is not linear. The route forward is up and down. Learning to be more flexible and being able to roll with things is a key skill. Life is uncertain by its very nature, meaning any discomfort with this presents a challenge. Becoming more adaptable means you will be able to see things for what they are, apply your best skills, and keep moving forward.

Knowing that there will be ups and downs allows you to prepare. You will be less surprised and be able to bring the right tools and practices online to address the circumstance. You only need to handle the moment in front of you right now, so what are your best options?

Drawing on your positive history, you can decide. These are life skills that will serve you well in overcoming your pain but also other challenges you will face. Many people taking this approach find that obstacles then become opportunities for learning.

Recharge points

When you make your daily plan, you can highlight your recharge points throughout the day. These are the times when you build or lift your energy.

There are many ways to manage your energy levels. They can include rest, reading, music, a shower, fresh air, meditation, movement, calling a friend, watching something funny or something else.

What are your ways of managing and boosting your energy?

Sometimes the recharge point will be longer than others. They can be a simple pause for 2-3 breaths, or perhaps 40 minutes of feet up and rest. Clarifying what you need and then making it a definite part of the day's schedule ensures you are doing this the best way. In time, as with other parts of your programme, you will adjust what you are doing and for how long.

If you make it part of your plan, you are more likely to follow through. Of course, it is your consistent actions that will make the difference to your quality of life.

Planning your day ties closely with habit formation. The Habits section will help you create new ones that create the conditions for the long-term transformation of your experiences. Each time you practise something, that is a vote for that version of you. It may not manifest immediately, but at some point in the future it will. What do you want that manifestation to look like?

Encouragement points

- Planning, prioritising, and periodising your day ensures that you get the important things done in the best way that you can, considering the circumstances.
- Having a plan includes recharge time, so you are actively managing your energy.
- Flexibility is needed because circumstances are always changing.
- You can review your plan and priorities to update your programme as you move forward.
- Sharing your plan means others know what you will be doing and perhaps how they can help.

Managing your expectations

'Undoubtedly, upstream of the things you do to get better is the ability to align expectations and reality.' RS

When you decide to do something new, you will have an expectation of what it will be like and how you will do it. Of course, this is all in the future, so it is guesswork. The future is always imagined. Your expectations arise from previous experiences and your beliefs about the world.

Your beliefs stem from the way you have been conditioned to think by people and the society in which you grew up. You were not born with them. Some higher beliefs (ones that you are not necessarily thinking about often but are hugely influential in your experiences) are installed from the beginning, such as the belief you will be cared for, loved, fed, and safety provided.

As a result, you have expectations about how the world operates, of yourself, how you should live, and those relating to each thing you do. You may not be overtly thinking about your expectations or being aware of them, but they are shaping your perceptions and experiences all the time.

In your mind you have an idea about what an activity will be like for you when you think about it. This happens automatically. In other words, you are not choosing how it looks because a thought pops in unbidden. These are automatic thoughts that you can become increasingly aware of with a meditation practice. With there being no choice in these thoughts arising, it is a matter of how you respond that makes the difference. There is also the question of whether this representation of the activity and situation is empowering or not.

If not, you can create another vision, one that empowers you to take action. Like self-awareness, this is a skill you can develop in order to keep on track.

If the activity is something you really want to be doing, you may have a strong desire to be there and doing it a particular way right now. But this may not be the reality, causing a mismatch. This can be frustrating and distracting because you are wanting to be somewhere other than where you are, resulting in suffering. The key is to be able to accept where you are right now and to focus on the next best step. This requires you to adjust your expectations in line with the reality of the circumstances.

Let's use walking as an example. You can apply this to any activity of course: for example, household chores, hoovering the lounge, getting out of bed, driving, going to the shop, climbing stairs.

Firstly, be clear about what you want to achieve: I want to walk _____ distance, choosing this according to your window of tolerance (either no or some symptoms, which have minimal impact and on balance you view the activity as a success). This is your vision and you are clarifying this by being realistic with your expectations.

The question you can ask yourself is: what can I do that is within my window of tolerance, considering the circumstances and how I am right now? This keeps you focused and accepting of where you are right now, maximising your chances of being successful. Creating your own opportunities for wins is a way to produce evidence that you can make progress and get better.

Other thoughts can appear of course. They could be in the form of unrealistic expectations (I should be able to …), the self-critic (I'm not good enough …), a fearful prediction (this will hurt …), a memory (last time I walked, it was agony …). They are all just thoughts that you are having. You are not those thoughts. They are real but often untrue. Becoming more self-aware, you realise this and become less entangled so you can refocus on what you are doing and what is really happening (being present).

You now have set a time or distance and are ready to go. There is no telling how it will go exactly. Uncertainty is life. However, you are doing your best and controlling what you can control: making a plan, keeping your expectations in line with reality, being in the right mindset, having the right attitude, and putting your energy into what you are doing. If you complete the distance, great! But this is just one aspect of the overall journey. You cannot control the outcome, only the effort you put in.

Sometimes you may not reach the target distance. If you measure your success solely on this outcome, you will feel that you have not done as well as you could. However, if you widen the lens and consider all the circumstances, you realise that sometimes despite your best efforts, the situation did not turn out the way you wanted it to. You can choose to measure success by doing it the best way you can.

Nature has its own plans and rhythm. The moment has gone, but you can find yourself clinging on to what has happened. The practice of acceptance helps you turn towards and be open to what happens, how it feels, your thoughts, and then, critically, let them pass by. This means you don't hold on for next time by adopting acceptance as a way of being. More on this later.

Part of you may expect to be pushing and forcing to make progress. This rarely if ever helps. In the short term, there may be a sense of gain, but then you have to bear the cost. This comes in the form of an increase in pain afterwards, which is not because of injury. Instead, it is because of an increased prediction of threat and a weighting towards prior experiences of pain over what is happening now biologically as a more reliable explanation for what is happening. Your reality has drifted away from the reality.

Consistently working this way will help you build your tolerance, confidence, and motivation as you gradually make your way towards your picture of success. It may seem counterintuitive if you believe that success only comes from pushing hard, but this typically results in an over-under-activity pattern with minimal progress, and much cost with a lot of frustration and feelings of failure. This is not necessary. Instead, we can focus on what works for you and build onwards.

Sharpening your axe

'Give me six hours to chop down a tree, and I will spend the first four sharpening the axe.' Abraham Lincoln

To get the most out of your practices and exercises, you need to prepare. The alternative is to allow things to happen by chance. I am sure you want better than that. You want the best results you can achieve.

Like many people, you may spend a lot of time on autopilot or in your head, instead of being present or connected with your body. Life can appear small and limited when mainly confined to the skull. There is another way.

To get results, you need to be present, focused, and attending to the details of what you are doing. You also need to be in the best state to practice or exercise.

You can also call this priming or getting into the zone. You sharpen your axe.

Preparation

People who want to perform at their peak, for example, athletes and musicians, will have a way of preparing or getting into the zone. They will have a routine that they use including thoughts, movements, or other cues. Watch a tennis player before he/she serves or a singer before going on stage and you will see.

You are no different. If you want to perform at your best, considering the circumstances, you must also have a way of being present and in the best state.

You will also need to be focused on what you want to achieve and do rather than what you don't. Whilst this sounds logical and simple, as humans we are very good at the latter. This is setting your intent and thinking about what you are going to do, and what you want to achieve.

Ways to prepare

Here are some ways you can set your intent and prime for the exercises you are about to practice.

1. The check in: how am I? What is happening for me right now? What is in my attention? Am I connected to my body?

Checking in is a key skill. By asking yourself these questions, you will answer them according to how you are now giving you an insight into what is actually happening, rather than the story you are telling yourself. These thoughts are always real, but are they true? That's the question to answer, which can only be done now, in this moment.

When you check in, it not only brings you to the present moment, the only one to handle, but also creates an opportunity to meet your needs or take action to get into a peak state.

During the day, checking in at regular points or when you switch tasks means you are consistently taking the opportunity to self-care, a vital part of overcoming pain.

Perhaps you have been sitting for a while and need some movement to nourish your body. You may need a drink, to deal with a matter causing you some anxiety or something else before you start practising. Then you will be able to focus.

2. How am I going to practice?

This is your intent. You can commit to practising in the best way in any given situation. Choosing to focus, be present and complete the expected repetitions will all point you in the right direction.

Creating your own mantra or cue can be helpful to get into the zone: for example, I will do my best, a triggering movement. Can you think of one?

3. Think about the movement you want to make

Rehearsing the movement or action prepares you more precisely. By choosing to focus on this purposefully, in effect you are then not focusing on other actions. This makes it more likely that you will move in the way you are rehearsing in your mind's eye.

This is called motor imagery. If you are a visual person, you will use imagery each day as a matter of course. When you think about dinner, for example, you may run a grainy kind of film in your mind's eye to decide what to eat and whether you need any groceries.

Some people think more in words and find imagery harder. Either way, we are setting our intent and thinking about what we want to do and how we want to do it.

There is similar activity in the brain when we are actively doing something and when we think about doing it. There is also activity when we watch someone else, meaning that we can understand what they are up to. Harnessing this is most useful in restoring normal, thoughtless movement.

Motor imagery is a powerful tool. It is used commonly by performers who want to get into the best state and be able to achieve peak performance: for example, musicians, athletes, and speakers. However, we can all use this technique to get the best results.

For instance, when you watch a penalty shootout, some of the players will be thinking about and imagining kicking the ball in a specific way into the goal. Then they execute the kick, which will be similar to the imagined version. If they become distracted by the crowd or more likely, a different thought (shall I kick it the other way?), this can affect the actual shot. Confused thinking affects movement.

Consider this for a movement you think will hurt. You want to reach out, but because of prior experiences, you think it will be painful. This is what you tell yourself. Often, this comes true as you know from your own experiences and from your new understanding of pain.

You become caught between wanting to perform the action and holding back, creating tension, altered movement, and error in the system (recall this is the difference between what is expected and what happens). Of course, the error is also an opportunity for learning, which is only possible when the fear is dealt with effectively. And the fear is dealt with by truly understanding your pain, hence this being the key first step.

What if you imagine reaching out in a smooth, confident way? When people practice this imagery, often they find that the actual movement is easier and less painful. It can be quite a surprise until they know why!

I encourage the use of imagery then actual movement, especially if it has been a challenge due to altered movements or pain (usually both). Think about what you want to do and how, then do it as best you can, stepping into those shoes.

4. Pause

Taking a moment before you practice allows you to be present and to focus. Without pausing, we just go from one thing to the next, the prior state informing us how we are now.

In your pause, you can take a few easy breaths to bring calm.

Preparing for your practices or exercises with more awareness and intent will improve the outcomes. It is not about getting them done and dusted—tick. It is about focus and quality to get the best results that you can, considering the circumstances.

Encouragement points

- Before you start practising or exercising, pause and check in: how am I?
- Think about the way you want to practise and why.
- Use imagery to activate your body systems that anticipate the action or movement you want to make.
- Pause between practices and refocus.
- Acknowledge your efforts and attitude.
- The key to best results is quality practice, repetition, and consistency.

Reconnection

'Much of the suffering comes from disengagement from what matters: people, purpose, the planet.' RS

Pain causes disconnection from what matters. We all have different things that are important to us in our lives, but there are some we have in common. I call them 3 Ps and a B. You may think of some other things that you want to reconnect with and use the strategies in this book to do so.

People

You are designed to connect to other people from the very beginning of your life. Your survival depends on it. In the early days of humans, to be banished from the group would mean huge risk to the individual who now must face the world alone. That would have been extremely dangerous and hence very threatening. This is one of the reasons why the feeling of shame is so powerful. Shame is triggered when there is a perceived social threat to your status or place in the group.

The fear of being rejected means that you behave in a way that ensures you stay connected to the group or an individual, whatever the cost. In the ideal world you receive unconditional love. You are accepted for who you are and loved regardless of your actions. Unfortunately, this does not always happen.

Children need unconditional love in particular. Early experiences of connection and touch are a normal part of healthy development. The relationships you form in your life are based upon what you have learned and the ways you have coped, making the early years important. Your idea of what a relationship should look like and how it should work is built in childhood and taken forward into adulthood.

Naturally there is great variance in people's beliefs about relationships because of different experiences. It goes without saying that they can be the basis for wellness as well as illness, the latter typically through chronic stress (see section on stress) from a difficult or abusive relationship. On the other hand, a healthy relationship can be enormously supportive and nourishing. In terms of pain, having a caring partner can make a difference to the intensity of the perception.

Ideally, you have people who inspire and encourage you. They see your strengths and support your growth as individuals. This could be a parent, a teacher, a coach, or someone else. Sadly, not everyone has encouragers in their life. There can be some very tough decisions to be made as to whether you should extract yourself from a relationship or environment that is not supporting your health and other needs.

The need for acceptance is innate and strong, meaning that you can put aside what matters to you or those things that bring health and wellness in exchange for fitting in. But at what cost? Understanding this allows you to make an informed decision.

Chronic pain often causes a withdrawal from social situations for a number of reasons. People tell me that they don't want to burden friends, that it is too difficult to go out or that they would rather stay in because it feels safer. There are many other reasons and the more that these are focused upon, the more likely the person will avoid such situations.

As well as staying at home more, there can be less contact with friends and family. If you have had to stop working, colleagues are also missed, together with those who you might spend time with playing sport or engaging in other social activities: for example, choirs, hobbies, clubs.

Loneliness is a big issue in society. Despite the opportunities to talk and communicate via devices, this is not the same as being in person. Even before the pandemic, loneliness had been identified as something society needed to address.

Researchers have known for some years that epigenetic changes occur when we *perceive* loneliness (Cole et al., 2007). Notice the word 'perceive'. It depends upon the person's own assessment of how connected they are in their life. You may know many people yet you feel lonely. On perceiving yourself to be lonely, your body systems switch to being pro-inflammatory. Inflammation is the beginning of the healing process but is also an underpinning biology for a sickness response and many common maladies such as depression and chronic pain.

From a survival (evolutionary) perspective, this makes sense. If you are isolated, you need your biology to be ready to heal your body if you are attacked by a lion. If you live in a group, it is more likely that you will transmit or receive a virus. The perception of being connected results in a more antiviral state, again making sense. So, inflammation at the right time and the right level is important and useful, whereas too much, prolonged, or at times when healing is not necessary, causes problems.

At a basic biological level then, we need to connect, especially for the sake of wellness. It also feels good in many cases. Think of a time when you were having a really good laugh with a friend. What do you notice right now, even at the thought? Laughter is at the essence of a great connection. Can you bring more humour into your life?

There is a feel to being connected with another person. This is a great state. The raw feelings will be personal to you. Again, bring a time when you were deeply engaged with someone you care about and notice how you feel now. The practice of bringing forth such imagery is a way to change state when necessary. You can then add movement and notice how this feels in a different, more relaxed state.

This in mind, it becomes important to reconnect with the people who matter in your life. Or, if you feel that the link is strong, you can build and strengthen the relationship. It could be argued that the quality of your relationships affects the quality of your life, emphasising their importance. At the heart of this is the value you place upon such relationships and your communication skills. Such skills can be practised and developed, having a positive effect on your relationships.

One skill is mindfulness, which helps you be present to really hear what the other person is saying. If you are present, you can listen deeply and truly understand their needs. Misunderstanding, on the other hand, often leads to conflict. Next time you are in conversation, you can try to be present and pay attention to what the other person is saying, resisting the temptation to interrupt or plan the next thing you want to say. Keep coming back to what is actually happening. You can then confirm what they have been saying and meaning by reflecting back in your own words, telling them what you have understood. This clarification not only tells them that you have been listening, but that you also care enough.

There are many ways that you can reconnect. You may already have some ideas. Here are some suggestions:

- Reach out to someone you have not spoken to in a while
- Send a text, expressing your gratitude for your friendship
- Even better, if you can, write a card or letter and send it
- Make a date to meet up
- Remind someone of a great time you had together
- Buy a gift for someone, for no particular reason

We can also choose to connect with people who we don't know. There is something interesting and positive about the fleeting exchanges we have in the shop or when buying a ticket. For instance, notice how the assistant responds when you ask them: how are you? It can be easy to miss these moments in the rush of life or if we are preoccupied.

Every encounter with another person is an opportunity to be curious (see section on curiosity), to be generous, to be compassionate, to practise listening, and to be energised. From a pain perspective, to connect in a positive way is to activate the affiliative system that is soothing. This is a felt experience you can note.

To know that someone who cares is present can make a significant difference to pain perception. Hand holding relieves pain for instance. Think about the child who is emotionally regulated by the loving act of a parent: a hug, a caress, a few kind words spoken with a soft voice. This can be equally important for an adult.

In a painful moment, we may just want a loved one to be there. They need not even say anything. There is an unseen yet felt connection. At the right time, they may offer help or a suggestion. This can help you to deal with the situation until you feel better.

On the occasion that you find yourself alone, you must self-soothe. This is a skill that you learn at a young age. For various reasons, some find this easier than others. Fortunately, you can develop and build this skill by practising certain techniques (see Self-soothing section) that can be used when needed. Like anything you practise, your ability and the effectiveness improve.

You may already understand the importance of both connections and the quality of these connections with other people and with ourselves. There is a tendency to set personal standards according to who you spend time with. You can bend to fit in and be part of the group. Whilst this is an advantage for people who are caring, compassionate, and live well, it also works the other way. Who you spend time with has an enormous effect on the quality of your life. This includes people who you watch, listen to, and whose words you read.

Purpose

Having a sense of purpose is what gets you up in the morning. There is something important and meaningful to do. This can be work, parenting, volunteering, exercising, or something else. Often, you have a number of purposes or things that you care about.

Suffering chronic pain can mean these activities are limited or have been curtailed. You may be off work or school or find it difficult to do what you used to. Many people avoid the jobs and tasks that they think will hurt or make things worse. Often this is based on a belief that pain equates to more damage or injury, but sometimes it is just the fear of the pain itself. This is the reason why we begin by making sure you understand your pain, address your fears, and help focus on the many ways you can move forward.

Losing your sense of purpose results in feeling listless and lost. Lacking motivation can manifest in different ways such as low energy levels, helplessness, and a search for the reasons why you feel bad that keep you stuck. This emphasises the importance of reconnecting with your purpose, which still exists. It never goes away, instead just getting lost in the undergrowth.

The first step is to clarify your purpose(s) by thinking about what matters to you in your life: for example, your family, your career, certain causes. Then you can connect with a time that you were engaged with your purpose: What was happening? What were you doing? How were you feeling? Who was there? What were you thinking? If you focus on this specific time, you will move into that state; a peak state.

In such a state, your mind will be more open to possibilities. Notice how your energy lifts. You did that, and you can do it again and again.

Secondly, you can be creative in the ways to take action. Here are a couple of examples.

- Parenting: if it is difficult and painful to care for young children, you may gradually reduce what you do with them. This is difficult for you as you want to be a good parent and it feels like the pain is stopping you from doing things the way you want to. The frustration and upset together with the pain can lead to you choosing to do less (e.g. bathing, carrying, hugging, playing), which in turn affects the way you feel about yourself. The focus is often upon what you and the kids are missing out on. One way to turn this around is by reconnecting with your purpose as a parent and then making a plan that you follow each day based on what you CAN do.
  - Why is it important to me to be a good parent?
  - What can I do right now to be a good parent?
  - What resources do I have?
  - What resources do I need?
- Work: chronic pain can affect your ability to work, which can be a time when you feel a sense of purpose. It is worth noting that currently the levels of engagement with work are low for a range of reasons. However, if you did feel that there was meaning in what you were doing and now can't work because of pain, this would be a disconnection from purpose. There are several ways to go about this.
- Clarify your purposes and start to engage with them step by step. These may relate to other areas of your life in the short term if you are unable to work, so that you can take immediate action (see below).
- If you cannot work, clarifying your purpose in relation to how you would like to be occupied and employed is a useful exercise. In so doing, you are starting to engage with a process of return to work, considering work in its broadest sense. Many people do resume work in which they can find some meaning. This is easier when you know your values and purpose.

- On your purpose being closer to the forefront of your thinking, you can make decisions based upon this and your values (see Values section). For example, your purpose may be to encourage others to achieve their best with what they do, or to serve others in such a way that their day and life is better. Although you may not yet be able to do this in the workplace, you can pursue this purpose in other ways, such as within your conversations with friends and family. You could set yourself a goal of having one encouraging chat each day and then build on having created a positive history.

Everyone has a purpose. Right now, you may not have it on the tip of your tongue. Both the busyness of life and suffering tend to obscure what matters and why, like an overgrown path in a forest.

You may remember a time when you were tired and suddenly felt energised by a friend suggesting that you do something together. Or when you felt down because something had happened to upset you, and in a flash you felt excited by a new thought that appeared without any bidding. These are changes in state and there are many ways you can do this by changing your focus, language, and moving your body.

In respect of reconnecting with a purpose, you can experience a boost that is enough to encourage and motivate you. Why? Simply because you are focusing on your intention and your reason for being, typically to serve something greater than the self. This lifts us, clears our thinking, and often illuminates a way forward. As mentioned above, this may need adapting to present circumstances, but nonetheless is a positive practice. Each step you take towards your picture of success is shaping something better in the future.

- *My purpose is …*
- *And …*
- *And …*
- *On reconnecting with my purpose, I feel …*

Planet (or nature)

When did you last take in a panoramic view across a valley, along a river, or out to sea? When did you last walk through a forest, lie on the grass, or tend to your garden? Or even think about a green space? I am talking about connecting with nature, which I call the planet to fit with the other Ps. Even if you live in a city, there will be green space, from a park to a window box.

Recently a study recommended two hours a week of being in nature because of the health-giving effects (White et al., 2019). It seems to be a simple suggestion that could benefit many. Further, nature is freely available.

In Japan, there is the practice of forest bathing called Shinrinyoku. You immerse yourself in the sights, sounds, feel, and smells of the trees, plants, and wildlife. Interestingly, it appears that essential oils released from trees (phytoncides) result in an increase in natural killer (NK) cells of the immune system (Li et al., 2010).

By nature, you can also think about the temperature of the environment, in particular cold. Most people in our society live in the comfort of a warm home and possess clothing to keep well insulated whilst outside in winter. They do not experience much in the way of discomfort due to cold. Yet cold can be a great daily therapy.

Not only can you build your ability to tolerate stress and discomfort with controlled cold exposure, but it also has a stimulating effect on the immune system. Some of this realisation has come from the work and practices of Wim Hof. Whilst you will find pictures of Wim swimming in icy lakes and running on snow bare-chested, there is a much more palatable practice: cold showers.

You may shudder at the thought initially. Most people I talk to tell me that they only take warm or hot showers. However, we can begin with our normal temperature and then gradually turn it down. With focus and breathing, you adapt to the cold. Thirty seconds to a minute will suffice before wrapping in a soft, warm towel if you wish. Otherwise, you can fully feel the effects in your own way, often energising. Cold therapy is not for everyone.

Although this is a simple practice, if you have any medical complaints or concerns, you should check with your doctor or healthcare provider.

Being in nature is a multi-sensory experience. We are bombarded with signals that our senses sample. Ultimately this results in a boost of wellness that we can often perceive as a feeling of greater energy and aliveness. It seems that this is especially the case in blue space, where there is water (White et al., 2020).

Not everyone has access to forests, lakes, and mountains, so here are some other suggestions:

- Take a walk in your local park
- Sit in your garden
- Stand or sit by a tree and look at its features

- Paddle in the sea (summer and winter)
- Plant some seeds and care for them
- Look at nature pictures on the internet
- Imagine being in nature, especially somewhere you know or have been before

Imagery and visualisation are powerful tools. When you imagine being somewhere, notice how you feel. Your body state changes, and you can start to embody the sensations as if you are actually there. On a more day-to-day basis, what happens when you are hungry and think about food?

Once you are in nature and immersed in what the planet offers, there are several practices you can use to get the most from your experience. The first is to turn off or silence your device to make it easier to be present. The second is to breathe in a relaxed way. Breathing is a useful way to be present as you oxygenate your body and activate the parasympathetic nervous system.

Access to nature can be a challenge if mobility is an issue or if pain limits how far you can walk or travel. This will require some creative thinking and perhaps help from a partner or friend. However, using the I CAN mindset, you think about what you could do with the resources that you have.

Further, you can view this as an opportunity to practise a certain level of activity upon which you can build. How you are now is not where you will be, and certainly not if you are practising shaping something better. Each choice you make now brings a different future. Keeping your eye on your picture of success is helpful. For more detail on how to make a plan, see the section: Bringing it together.

- *What opportunities do you have to immerse yourself in nature each week?*
- *What will you definitely do each week? And when?*
- *What help will you need?*

Body

You are a whole person. What does this mean?

It means you are thinking, feeling, moving human being in the world, as perceived by you. However, the wholeness refers to the one experience that you are having right now. Your thoughts are not separate from your body and the way that you move is not distinct from how you perceive yourself in the environment you are in.

In fact, our experiences that unfold each moment are where thought, action, and perception meet. And there is nothing you have to do to make these things happen. The fact that you are conscious means that your awareness is full of thoughts, sights, sounds, smells, feelings, emotions, attitudes, and more. There is a constant stream of contents all appearing in the same place. You can become more familiar with this through meditation.

Why is this important to know? Simply because we have been told for many years that mind and body are somehow separate. Our healthcare and social systems are based on this division. We have hospitals and departments for body parts and another building over the road for the mind. But that is not how we work or experience ourselves.

There has been a raft of fascinating research and work over the years looking at how we think, act, and perceive from the perspective of an embodied mind (Varela, Thompson & Rosch, 2017). This field has a long history in philosophy and now much data supporting the notion that the mind is embodied. You think the way you do because of the body that you have. Your body state is influencing how you think and the types of decisions that you make. What you are thinking about is affecting your body state. It all comes together. Yet you can have a say in what happens next by becoming more self-aware and using the types of practices and tools suggested in this book.

In particular, some scientists have been studying interoception to deepen our understanding (Tsakiris & De Preester, 2018). They have discovered many fascinating findings that are relevant to how we think about pain and consequently how we can address pain in better ways. Interoception is the sense of our internal physiology, such as our heart beating and gut rumbling.

It is thought that these feelings sensed inside your body contain messages for you to act in order to manage your metabolism and ultimately your ongoing existence. We can go a stage further and consider that all thoughts, feelings, and sensations that we perceive are in service of keeping our biology within certain parameters for survival. This is a priority, of course, and probably one of the reasons why pain is such a big deal. It is meant to be.

Under normal, healthy circumstances you feel a sense of wholeness. You are aware of your body, albeit in a transparent way, and typically not thinking about it too often. Pioneering physiotherapist Louis Gifford spoke of thoughtless and effortless movement, which strikes of being in flow. This is a challenge when you are suffering pain because the body is the source of suffering, and despite what we know about pain as a perception, it has a quality of physicalness.

Your body systems are generating your experience of pain, weighing up current sensory information in the light of past experiences. It is unique to you and to that moment. Your pain is different from my pain, and I can never know what yours feels like. So, when someone says, I can feel your pain… they can't. Of course, no one can actually feel someone else's pain. It is possible to feel pain in your body when another person speaks of theirs, which is a form of empathy. I am often aware of my body in the same location that the person sitting opposite me is describing. On the plus side, this gives me some appreciation and allows me to bond on a deeper level.

Pain is not just about what is happening now. You will recall from the Understand Pain section that the brain is part of the orchestra of your body systems that make predictions. So when you feel and think something, this is a prediction to best explain the current circumstances (e.g. your biology, situation) and is in anticipation of what could happen next. You predict your needs and mobilise resources accordingly. For instance, before standing up, your body systems predict this action, what it will be like and what is needed. Blood pressure goes up before standing therefore, otherwise it would be too late, causing errors in the system felt as light-headedness or dizziness.

Pain being about a perceived threat, there may not actually be anything dangerous happening right now, but there could be in the near future. This assessment is more likely if there have been repeated pain episodes that are now priors informing the present moment. Hence, persisting pain (not constant—this is not possible) makes persisting pain more likely until the predictions are updated. Prediction updating is what you are seeking to achieve with your tools and practices. There is nothing wrong with the prediction machinery so to speak, but the predictions themselves are not a very good representation of what is actually happening. Your grip on the world has drifted, which is not a conscious effort by the way. You are certainly not doing this on purpose.

This in mind, predicting that there could be a threat based on what you know and have experienced before, pain could be the best explanation. The problem with many cases of chronic pain is that the predicted experience of pain is real. It is your reality. But is it not a good representation of the reality, which is that your body is healthier than it may feel. There is no actual threat to your integrity as a whole. This understanding is important because you can see why and how you can feel pain in absence of any tissue damage or pathology. In turn, this allows you to reassure yourself, self-soothe and decide on your next best action, which could be to return to what you are doing.

A further example of using anxiety may help to clarify.

You have to give a public talk. When thinking about standing in front of a group of people, you feel anxious. But you are not actually in that room. You are in your lounge, watching TV. Suddenly the thought pops into your awareness, even though a moment ago you were relaxed. You did not choose to think about the talk, the grainy image or words simply appeared. Now you feel very different inside, despite the outside world changing only very slightly (recall impermanence).

On the basis that you will be giving that talk, your brain begins to budget for this and mobilises resources, including those that arise as feelings of fear or worry. Whilst this is not a feeling that you like, it can be useful as it motivates you to prepare in order to do your best job. It is a normal and necessary feeling.

So, the way that your body feels informs your thinking and actions. The decisions that you make are determined by your body state. When you are tired, everything can feel like an effort. Just the thought of going to the shop to get some milk feels tiring. But your state can change depending on what you do with your bodies and thoughts. You have far more control than you might believe. I hope that you gain a sense of this once you have read this book and started practising changing state.

Back to the importance of connecting with the body. It is both understandable and protective to somehow detach from the body if it is deemed to be a source of suffering. You start doing this early in life. Think of a young child having a temper tantrum as they experience all these strong feelings and emotions, but without any understanding, trying to get away from them.

In more frightening circumstances, you can fully dissociate and sometimes see yourself from an out-of-body perspective. This is a feature of trauma and there are many shades of intensity. Most people will have a dissociative experience in their life due to stress, tiredness, drugs, or alcohol. In some people, the feeling sticks and they repeatedly dissociate, often causing much distress until they understand what is happening.

It can be peculiar and hard to describe, causing many people to keep it to themselves and suffer in silence. There is certainly a compromise of the sense of wholeness. Dissociative disorders (DPD) come in different forms. Depersonalisation is one form that feels like you are outside your experiences and derealisation another, when the world feels unreal as if there is some kind of veil between you and it. People describe it in many different ways.

There is some excellent work being done to understand DPD (Ciaunica & Charlton, 2018). If you think that this is something you experience, it is important to talk to a clinician who understands the condition.

A change in body sense is common in persistent pain. Certainly, it can be a feature of complex regional pain syndrome (CRPS), a terribly painful condition. People will often describe how the affected limb feels detached, that it is not theirs or a different size. I ask the question routinely and encourage people to tell me about all of their perceptions.

This creates the opportunity to explain what is happening and ease fears. Many have not told their prior therapists and doctors for fear of feeling foolish despite this being a really important part of the picture. Normalising body sense is a key part of getting better as you will see.

On another level, the body area that hurts can often be grabbing attention, relentlessly in some cases. Why would you want to connect with such pain when you just want it to go away? If pain like this compels one thing, it is the desire for relief. When you find it hard to self-soothe or do something to feel better, somehow trying to get away from your body may seem like a good idea.

But it's not an active choice. You cannot decide to change the way you sense your body or whether you are connected to it in a moment of suffering. It just happens. However, you can decide what to do next, and this might be to turn your attention towards the pain and how you are feeling about it in order to transform your suffering. This is something you can work towards being able to achieve as you can only overcome pain by facing it and changing your relationship and responses (see Challenging moments).

Or as it stands, you may have another way of coping in the moment if the intensity of the pain is severe. In fact, you will do whatever comes to mind. The key point is that if you are practicing skills to deal with difficult moments as a matter of day-to-day training, you will get better at using them when you need to.

We live in a society that often encourages you to distract or ignore your own suffering. You may have been taught that any kind of self-care is selfish and indulgent. Yet the fact remains that to overcome pain means you must care for yourself. Building these skills is vital for your own wellness and your ability to contribute to those around you and society.

Practically, there will be times when turning towards the reasons for your suffering are easier (not easy, but easier!) and others when the intensity of the pain will require survival of those moments. You are training yourself to manage challenging moments more skilfully and be able to increasingly self-soothe, reassure, create calm, and then make your next best decision: how can I create the conditions to feel better? This is in service of learning and moving forward.

Reconnecting with the body comes in different forms, commonly with movement. Certainly, this is encouraged as a way to overcome trauma, often blended with psychotherapy (van der Kolk, 2014). People practise yoga, Pilates, walking, breathing, mindfulness, and other activities to become increasingly aware of their bodies as a means to reconnecting and feeling whole. The sense of the body becomes more familiar, which is essentially transparent.

When I talk about the sense of the body, I am referring to the feeling of knowing where you are in space and in relation to the environment. You may have heard the term proprioception to describe it. An accurate sense means that you can walk around furniture, through doorways, and pick things up with precision. Think about writing, doing up buttons, or typing on a phone. It is easy to take this for granted as you do not normally have to think about where you are, unless it is dark, you are somewhere unfamiliar, or perhaps on uneven ground. Many people tell me that they have become clumsy, bumping into furniture, and dropping things. This can be a sign that body sense has become blurry. Another way to put it is that movement is less precise and economical. Refined movements become more gross, using extra muscle power. Sharpening the precision of movement is an important part of getting better as you will see.

If you have pain or anticipate that a movement will hurt, the body is very much in your awareness. It is like the difference between looking through a window forgetting that there is a glass pane because you see just the view, and noticing a crack. The view is now obscured. Then there are other competing considerations in the form of your thoughts. Can you do it (the chosen activity/task)? Will it hurt? How much will it hurt? Will you be able to sit in that chair? And so on.

All this extra chatter, analysis, judgement, expectation, and anticipation actually take you away from the present moment. Whilst you cannot stop this chatter that feels so real, accompanied by echoes in the body as felt sensations, you can become increasingly present so you can notice and respond skilfully rather than on autopilot. The chatter is another crack in the window, separating you from what is really happening in the world. Pausing, perhaps using your breathing practice (see this section), helps you to see the thoughts for what they are as you make your next best decision, bringing back clarity and presence.

Developing precise and economical movement to the point where it is transparent once more is a goal. The reason you move is to achieve certain goals depending on what you need and what is available in the environment (affordances). From an embodied cognition perspective, you move to perceive. In other words, the way you move and the range of movements you are able to enact will create your perceptions of the world. This is why being limited or anticipating that there will be pain affects the way you experience both yourself and what is around you.

Normalising body sense and movement come hand in hand and beget each other. Often confidence in yourself and your body grows as movement becomes easier and more thoughtless. People often notice how they have more energy as conscious anticipation lessens and how they are just doing, without so much thought. Flow resumes, intermittently at first, as you move towards greater freedom.

Encouragement points

- Reconnecting with what matters is an important part of improving your life and overcoming pain.
- In particular, reconnecting with people, a purpose, the planet, and your body.
- There are practical ways of doing this that are part of your programme.
- Making this a conscious practice when you are aware of how it feels to reconnect takes you to the heart of a whole-person approach.

Ups and downs

'Understanding and overcoming pain is an up and down journey. A dimly lit path. Because life is up and down and uncertain. Let's shine a light on the way forward.' RS

There is no straight, upward line of recovery. Instead, there will be ups and downs. That is normal, as life is up and down, with each moment being different and new.

Accepting this reality is vital. Otherwise, you are met with regular disappointment, frustration, and perhaps a sense of failure. This can become your story, which is one of doing worse than you expect and want. But this is another story that you can come to see is holding you back. This is not an actual failure. It is resistance to what is, usually accompanied by unrealistic expectations. Both you can deal with effectively, but better at the outset, and not once we have started down the bumpy track.

There is an argument that whenever you feel resistance, it is because something is hitting your belief system. This is a useful way to think about it and a practical way of knowing your current position relative to where you seek to go.

There are many examples of resistance in our lives. Some big and some small. Nonetheless, they are there day in and day out, affecting the way you feel, often subconsciously. For instance, you could resist the weather because your preference is for sunshine. Or you may resist the fact that you cannot sit for as long as you want to. Perhaps you can think of some other examples.

What does resistance achieve? When you resist, it feels bad. There can be tension, stress, irritation, annoyance, frustration, and more. Does this change the circumstances? Does your resistance to the situation do anything to it? Of course not. And you know this, yet continue to resist, clinging to the belief that it should be a different way.

On the other hand, when you practise acceptance (see later section), the resistance dissolves, making freedom possible. It also means that you are able to see things as they are and deal with them in the most skilful manner. How does that sound to you?

Why are there ups and downs in getting better? Simply because life is full of them. The way you are feeling changes throughout each day. Sit for just a few moments and notice how many different thoughts and feelings you experience. They come. They go. That is normal.

The issue comes in how you relate to your thoughts and how you respond, not the thoughts themselves. Fortunately, this is a skill you can develop. Do you cling to certain ideas about the world and yourself? For instance, do you cling to the idea that you have to do things perfectly? Or look a particular way to be accepted? Clinging like this causes stress, disturbing inner peace, and often worsening pain.

Sometimes you have an idea why you feel the way that you do, and at other times you don't, so you guess. This becomes your story; your reality. But often it is not the reality. Life is happening regardless of your or anyone's preferences or desires. Life is happening. There is a reality going on. Life is really there, and so are you. But you have a version of this going on, being generated by your body systems. It is your reality but not the reality. This is a vital insight. You don't directly experience life, which is why sometimes you can drift far from the reality in your thoughts. Thoughts are real (they feel so real!) but how true are they? Is that thing you are thinking about actually happening?

Being able to see thoughts for what they really are and to be open to other possibilities is a useful skill. You are not ignoring your thoughts and feelings. It is important to recognise them and acknowledge how you are feeling. Then you can check in on what is actually happening for you before choosing the next best action that is in line with your picture of success and according to what matters to you in life (value-based decisions).

What is your next best decision?

We can deal with the ups and downs by learning to ride the waves rather than trying to force through them. An influential book by philosopher Andy Clark captures this nicely with the title Surfing Uncertainty. Life is full of uncertainty— fact. Life is only possible because of uncertainty. Things are always changing as no moment is ever the same. You can embrace this as part of the adventure, or at least learn how to cope with this fact better and better. Fighting uncertainty causes suffering because you are fighting and resisting life that is happening anyway, regardless of what you like or do not like.

So how can you minimise the impact? What skills can you learn and what approach can you take? How can you best think about the challenges as they arise? These are all useful questions. I hope you will start to have some answers as you read and finish this book. Maybe you have some already to note down.

Different traditions offer ways. Buddhism and Stoicism form the basis for ways to live life by recognising certain facts and then dealing with them skilfully. Does that sound like a good idea to you? If you are interested in going deeper, you can go back to the original sources such as the Dhammapada or the writings of Seneca and Marcus Aurelius.

When we can see and understand the nature of things as they really are, as opposed to our biased thinking and interpretation, there is an opportunity to learn and move forward. This is the case even if there is discomfort. A phrase that is often heard is becoming comfortable with the uncomfortable. It means that we can train ourselves to be fine with the fact that there is going to be some kind of suffering on a day-to-day basis. Buddhism has always acknowledged that life is full of suffering, but that there are ways we can relieve our suffering by following a particular path. This path is determined by the teachings and practices that we can all access.

This is true for us who lead modern lives. Thich Nhat Hanh, a Vietnamese Buddhist monk who has been hugely influential through his teachings and writings, speaks of engaged Buddhism. This is an approach for the likes of you and I who do not desire to become monks or nuns but do wish to learn practical skills to improve our lives.

At this point, I would like to say that I am not encouraging you to follow a particular spiritual path. That is entirely your choice. My suggestion is to become familiar with and skilled at using particular practices that can relieve your suffering. It may sound somewhat mystical; however, there has been a great deal of research looking at what happens when we meditate, cultivate compassion, and are mindful. This work is ongoing and extremely encouraging, together with reported experiences.

The most common bump in the road is called the flare up. This is when the pain feels worse. Sometimes this is after doing a particular activity, something new or different, or on occasion without any obvious cause. Remember the varied relationship of cause and effect and that there are always surrounding variables that we have no access to or knowledge of. We may have a sense of something that contributed, and we would be wise to consider this in our next steps. Perhaps we choose to moderate the movement or be more exploratory and curious.

One of the challenges is that a particular stimulus at a point in time may not manifest as an experience for some time afterwards. This could be hours, days, weeks, or even months. The reason is within our biology. I don't like to reduce things, but for convenience consider the changes in form and function in the nervous system, particularly if there is nerve damage causing neuropathic pain. The change in the neuron triggered by the stimulus, when the proteins are created and passed down the axon to the terminal, takes a variable amount of time. This explains the latent effect. I did something on Monday, and the pain was worse on Saturday.

When the person tells their story at the outset, we must listen carefully. There may have been an episode of back pain that seemed to resolve after a few weeks. Then, several months later, leg symptoms began: pins and needles, some pain in various locations down the limb, a different sense of the leg and perhaps some mild weakness. This latter presentation was brewing from the start but took some time to become an experience. The two seemingly different stories are actually one. Our role as clinicians who understand the biology of pain must be able to help you understand what has happened before looking at what to do next.

What is the best way to manage a flare up? As they are part of the way forward, this is an important skill set to learn and develop. Perhaps it is a useful way to think about flare ups: an opportunity, albeit unpleasant. We don't want the experience, but it is inevitable, hence acceptance being important. And acceptance does not mean giving in or giving up. It means that we recognise and admit where we are within the bigger picture of our lives. It will also be important to remember impermanence, considering that however we are feeling right now, it will change in time.

It may seem sensible to try and avoid flare ups by playing it safe. We can create a set of rules that we follow in order to stay within certain parameters. This is a list of dos and don'ts, cans and can'ts. Another way to put it is limitations and avoidances. In the short term, avoiding particular movements or activities means that I don't feel the anticipated pain and instead feel safe. Familiar?

The problem arises when we realise that life is not static and that things are always changing. Those rules will stay the same, but we do not, despite this feeling of sameness—it's the same me. Hence the limits and avoidances become harder and narrow further. Life becomes more restricted and so on. The opposite way, facing and seeking to transform our pain can seem challenging, overwhelming, and largely unappealing. Yet this is the route towards what we want our lives to be like, defined by an increasing freedom of choice. We want to be able to take opportunities in a given environment rather than avoid them.

To do this takes courage, perseverance, and patience. But you have all those, so how do you use them? What are the practical steps to take?

Firstly, we create our new habits and routine that form the day-to-day practices and exercises, interwoven into our life—they are part of the day, not separate. Consistency helps to flatten the curves of uncertainty and moves us away from a tendency for over- and under-activity cycles. However, despite these efforts, flare-ups happen. As I intimated before, perhaps these have some use in terms of learning, despite their unpleasantness or even vileness at times.

Secondly, we can prepare. For this, we can draw upon the ways that people rehearse for stressful situations so that when they arise, they can perform certain skills in a calmer and more focused way. An example would be a firefighter or another professional emergency role that requires clear thinking and responses over reactions and panic. There is not an exact comparison as pain is extremely personal and an urgent in the compulsion to get relief in some cases, yet the skills are useful.

Some of the consistent practices that bring calm and perspective are those that become increasingly effective when there is a need. There is something about a daily practice or practices throughout the day that translates into one's overall approach. Greater clarity of thought and skilled action emerge from practice. There may come a time when such a practice, for example, breathing (see relevant section), is one of the go-to skills at a time when triggers are noticed or during a painful moment.

Just as you can rehearse for a part in a play, you can rehearse what you will say to yourself and the action you will take at a time when you are challenged by an increase in pain. A new script, breathing, certain movements, moving your attention, and listening to music are all examples of things you can do to change your state. In essence, this is what you are trying to do—change state biologically and experientially; the two have some relation. I encourage people to create a list of resources that they can call upon at challenging times: what kinds of things can I do to feel better?

An important point at this time is to recognise that what we do may not have an immediate effect. Where we set our expectations plays a role in how successful we feel that we have been and whether we continue. Knowing that we are taking positive action in line with our picture of success can help, but so does realising that we may have to combine different practices or be patient in how things change, which they will. This removes the pressure and consequent frustration or stress that only adds to the very feelings we are trying to resolve. Again, this is not necessarily easy, but is it possible. And we do get better as we practise because they are skills, which can also give some encouragement.

Create your flare up plan then, before it happens. You can update what you do as your skills develop and you realise what works best for you.

Encouragement points

- Recovery is not linear. Instead, reflective of life, it is an up and down journey.
- Knowing this means we can prepare and keep our expectations in line with reality.
- Flare ups are when there is a temporary increase in symptoms, which you can learn to manage skilfully.
- Practicing skills at calmer times means that you will be able to use them more effectively when needed.
- You can create a plan for when you need to use such skills.

Self-soothing

'We have or can learn and develop a powerful ability to self-soothe, which is an important skill in tricky moments.' RS

Self-soothing is the ability to look after yourself when you need to calm and feel better. This is no different from when you want to help someone you care about, except you are turning your compassion towards yourself. There are different ways that you can do it.

Self-soothing is something you learn early in life by observing and experiencing the way that others soothe you and learning how it feels. Sadly, some people don't have these experiences, meaning that self-caring is a challenge. However, they are skills that you can learn and develop at any age, although they may feel strange or uncomfortable to begin with.

Another way to think about it is to be able to apply the brakes when we notice the triggers or cues to stress, pain, or other states. Pema Chödron talks of hooks—those moments when we feel tension or other feelings in the body before it becomes a full-blown experience. Becoming increasingly skilful at recognising your hooks means you can self-soothe or apply the brakes and be able to navigate the feelings and situation.

For instance, you may come to understand that the way a particular person says certain things brings up a feeling of anger and tension. Knowing this and being aware of the beginnings of bodily changes enables you to see what is happening and practise responding in a different way. In turn you have a different experience, hopefully better, which you build upon. Cultivating this self-awareness is one of the effects of regular mindful practice (see Mindfulness).

There are times when self-soothing can be a useful tool when you are suffering pain at a given moment. This is one of the ways you can learn to respond rather than react. The implication to yourself is that you are in more control, feeling empowered to take action. So, what actions can you take?

Before coming to these, it may be useful to think about what taking a different action actually does for you.

In addition to feeling that there is something you can do, as opposed to feeling helpless, taking action is a fundamental way of getting better. How so? By choosing to do something that makes sense to you as a useful tool, you gain a knowing and an expectation that you are more and more in the driving seat. Naturally this can vary. Some days are just harder than others. But if you can keep practising as consistently as you can, then you increasingly know that you are heading in the right direction.

Some people start to feel better on this basis. But not always. Here's the paradox. The more you do things with the thought in mind that you are doing it to achieve a certain endpoint, often the more distracted you are from doing the very thing that can help. The skill lies in being focused on the step you are taking right now. This is about being present and creating the conditions for a better future—immediate and sustained. Again, mindfulness practice is useful for learning to be present and focus on the process over the prize. The latter comes from attending to the former (see Process over prize).

To take a different action means that you will get different results in time. How that turns out depends on your ability to notice what is really happening versus a story that may be saying something else—we tell ourselves things that appear to be utterly compelling. It works the same the other way around. To keep reacting the same way will tend to mean we experience the ongoing suffering as we did before. The caveat is impermanence of course. Nothing ever actually stays the same as each moment is fresh and new. What can stay the same is the story and telling ourselves that nothing has changed. That in itself is something interesting to explore: why would we continue to believe that things are the same when they are not?

Perhaps one explanation is that our sense of self usually remains somewhat the same—it feels like 'me' now as it always did. This stability is important to regulate our biology, which has only one purpose. To survive. So, to create that sense of stability, we tend towards believing that things are the same because the opposite would be uncertainty, which is harder to handle despite this being a feature of life.

For different reasons, some people need certainty. This is something that has developed through social conditioning and experiences to date, so there is no blame attached. You have been shaped by both of these together with your genes when you did not choose your mind in the first place. You did not choose to be you. This is an important realisation when it comes to working with the self-critic through the lens of compassion. You did not choose to exist or to be you. But now you have had this insight, you can take responsibility for the way that you go about living and thinking. This is work of course, but worthwhile I would argue, in terms of improving your life and reducing suffering.

Back to the need for certainty, this poses a problem because there are only a few things you can control: for example, our attitude, intent, approach, and some actions. You cannot control others or the world despite your efforts or beliefs. Yet many try and fail, resulting in frustration or more self-criticism; essentially more suffering. Learning to focus on what you can control then becomes a key life skill and one that is vital for overcoming pain. It is also, I would argue, a way of self-soothing.

By thinking about what I can control and do in a given situation means that I am doing my best. This is all you can do. Anything beyond that is unrealistic or unfair to yourself. This is easier said than done of course, as people often set their expectations of themselves too high or a part of them tells them that they should be able to do certain things, despite them being out of line with what they want to achieve (see Expectations).

The more immediate self-soothing practices that I often suggest to people I am working with are low tech, and therefore available in most situations. They change our state biologically and experientially. Initially you recognise that you are in a particular state, for example, pain or anxiety. Then you acknowledge and accept what is happening at that moment. This is rather than resisting, which only leads to more suffering (although we are pretty good at resisting what is!). Next, you can consider the circumstances and notice what is happening for you. Finally, you choose the best action: what is my best decision now? And now?

There are a couple of important points raised here: noticing what is happening and considering the circumstances. Both rely on you being present and able to look from a distance rather than being caught up. Creating that space is a skill in itself and one that emerges from mindfulness. This space helps you see things for what they are and make a good decision rather than being carried along with the waves of emotion.

As with all practices though, sometimes we will be better than others. Accepting this as normal is important and helpful. You are doing your best with what you have at this moment. Afterwards, you can reflect and learn—What worked and what did not? What did I do well and what could I manage or do better next time?

To consider the circumstances gives you the opportunity to understand why things work differently at different times. With time ever moving forward, there is constant change afoot, although you may not feel or realise it. Impermanence makes life possible. There is no one single constant state that you are in. So, when you use a skill, you can be aware of the circumstances to give perspective and see the bigger picture. Zooming out in this way can be most helpful.

For example, I may decide to walk a certain distance, say one mile. This is my goal or target. I expect to be able to do this and set off. About halfway I start thinking that maybe I need to turn back because of pain or some other concern. Part of me says I must keep going because that is the goal and the only measure of success. In other words, if I don't complete the mile, I have failed, or even stronger, I am a failure. Another part of me, the self-caring and compassionate part, says it is ok because you are doing your best, considering the circumstances. What are the circumstances? I had a disturbed night, which made me more sensitive, and there were some stressful situations at home this morning. This will inevitably affect your performance.

Setting the bar of success so that doing your best is the achievement changes everything. You self-soothe by understanding the situation fully, then make your best decision, which on this occasion could be to walk half a mile. There are always ups and downs. But by working with yourself rather than against yourself and pushing at the wrong times, you will gradually increase what you are doing over a longer period and in a sustained way. The short-term satisfaction of keeping going for the mile may meet the need of one part of you but then you suffer the consequences. An increase in symptoms having pushed is the cost and now when you come to the next practice, this prior experience plays an informative role. Remember the key principle of having good and positive experiences that you curate action and build upon.

On completing the walk, acknowledging the success of doing the important thing (walking) and doing it the best way that you could (considering the circumstances), results in a good experience for the next time. Conversely, if you push through and flare up, this will inform the next effort, reinforcing the story that walking is painful instead of something I can do and build upon. The latter is what we consistently aim for as you move forward on your journey of reconnecting with what matters.

Each step along the way as you think about what you are going to do, see the bigger picture within which you are acting, and making decisions can be done in the light of self-soothing.

Self-soothing, then, is an approach fostering compassion and practical wisdom. The aim is to be in the best states as often as possible so that you can make choices in line with building the future life you want. It encompasses calming, rationalising, dampening down, easing from a reaction to a skilled response, gentle nudging in a particular direction, and caring about yourself.

People often tell me that this is an alien feeling or practice. The main reason given is because it is self-indulgent or selfish. You have been brought up to put others first and to believe that self-caring is ego-driven. The idea of me time has been popularised and usually means a period when you choose what you do, typically something pleasurable or meaningful. This is an interesting concept because we are with ourselves all of the time anyway. What is really meant is there is a need to be seen and acknowledged as a person who has desires to be fulfilled, and this is when I will do it—me time.

When it comes to self-caring, the usual explanation is that to look after others in the way that you want, you must look after yourself. This makes sense, but does it happen for you? As with most of the practices and tools, it is about grooving a habit (see Habits). You may start with a short break when you do something you enjoy for a few moments. When you have been successful, you then add other times to build momentum and the effects across the day and your life.

I would argue that to self-soothe well, you need to be able to self-care, which is why I raise the point. The two seem to sit together, with some overlap in the practicalities: the focus on self, time, and intent.

There are three self-soothing practices that are available to you at anytime and anywhere. These are tools at the top of the box, ready. They are breathing, touching, and moving. Of course, as you become more skilful, you can use them together in different combinations. On using them, if you are paying attention, you will feel the change in state (even subtle), which can be layered upon with further practices to keep going in a particular direction.

Again, I bring up your expectations. If you start using a practice and you are expecting it to work 100%, and this only means complete pain relief or cessation of anxiety, you are likely to feel disappointed and perhaps a failure. The knock-on effect can then be telling yourself that the practice does not work, and you stop. This is often an error. Not because of what you have done, but in setting expectations at the wrong level and focusing on prize over process. I probably talk about this more than anything else because it lies at the heart of getting better or not.

Helpful to understand this, although not necessarily popular, is that there is a time factor. Choosing a particular action or set of actions does not necessarily bring about immediate change that is desired. Instead, it is knowing that you have taken a positive step, which in itself can make us feel better through empowerment, and that you are heading in the right direction as best you can. Considering the circumstances and what you have available to you.

Self-soothing practice: Breathing

The first and commonly used practice is breathing (see Breathing). In my view this is an underused and underrated practice by many, when in fact it is one of the most potent ways of changing state. There are many ways to breathe.

In the situation where you want to self-soothe, there are two ways I suggest. There are others you may discover as well of course.

Some people find that slowing their breathing for a few breaths creates a pause and some space to make the next best decision. Or to be able to see things for what they really are in that moment. This can take several different forms. I encourage you, if you can, to use your nose for breathing. Why? Because your nose is for breathing and you know now because you have read the Breathing section.

1. Count to 4 as you breathe in, count to 4 as you breathe out. Repeat x 2-3. You can continue if you like, to create deeper calm, gain a sense of control and feel the change in chemistry inside. Some people find 4 hard, so you can shorten the counting. You can also extend it to 5/5 or 6/6. These numbers bring your breathing rate down to 5-6 breaths per minute, changing your state and creating evidence that you can be calmer and at peace.

2. Breathing awareness: this is a practice suggested by Thich Nhat Hanh and his community. In a way, this is a less technical form of breathing, 'only' requiring you to become aware of your breathing as it is and to follow the sensations as they appear and change. You simply observe your breath as your breathe in, and as you breathe out. When your mind wanders, you begin again. People often think they have done it wrong when they become lost in thoughts. This is normal. Starting again is part of the practice. Often as a result of sitting back and observing, you slip naturally into a calm and relaxed state when your body systems are then able to do all their healthy work.

Both of these practices require our attention, and in turn by practising you are also improving your ability to focus (see Focus and attention). Inevitably your mind will wander at some point. This is normal and fine. It is an opportunity to recognise that it has happened and to return your attention to the sensations of breathing. You can think of this as a rep, as in repetitions of an exercise. More reps equal more practice and learning. In this light, there is no such thing as a bad practice. Only success or learning.

Self-soothing: Touch

Many people find touch (see Touch) to be soothing. It can also be a challenge for different reasons. Bad experiences of touch in the past can have an ongoing effect. Some people are sensitive to touch for neurodevelopment or social reasons. Those suffering from persistent pain can find touch difficult because of the neuroimmune changes and the predictions of pain under certain circumstances that involve contact. For example, a light touch that results in a pain experience is called allodynia (pain due to a stimulus that does not normally provoke pain).

This happens because the brain predicts that the sensory information is best explained by pain, despite the signals in the periphery being initiated by light touch receptors. The modulation of the signals as they travel up the system, being predicted all the way through the different levels of the neuroimmune system, means that they can blend with danger signals. However, you will recall that even with these signals, the brain will still make its best guess by weighting either prior experiences or sense data. It is not a given that we feel pain just because of certain signals from the body.

This is important background, and you may like to review the pain section to deepen your understanding. Your experiences are always changing and are different. Having insights into how and why this can happen helps you make the best decisions, and also highlights the importance of consistency and hitting the right levels of practice.

The specifics of touch are described in that section. The purpose of using touch to self-soothe is the same as if you were to show caring for another person. What would you do? You may put a hand on their back or shoulder. Or perhaps light stroking, which stimulates specific nerve endings that only respond to this kind of touch. It is a system that has been well studied and enables us to bond. Just as the action is a clear demonstration to another, it is a clear demonstration to yourself that you care, you are worthy of such care, and changes your state.

A further type of touch is mild pressure massage. This is felt but not so much that it evokes a guarded response (e.g. flinching or tensing). Essentially, you want it to be a pleasant, nourishing experience. This level of touch appears to stimulate the parasympathetic nervous system, which is why we can feel a sense of ease and calm.

However, this is not always possible depending on the level of sensitivity in that moment. If some pain is inevitable, then it is important to work within the window of tolerance. This means that you are having a positive experience on balance, which you have created by deciding how to touch and for how long.

Self-soothing: Movement

This may be surprising to consider as often movement is painful. Yet there are different types of movement and ways to use it. You can also move your body away from the sensitive area and gradually work towards it.

Movement (see Movement) is fundamental for your health and wellness. Also to take the opportunities that the environment offers. There is not much we can achieve without movement. Including creating our own perceptions, which are informed by the movements themselves.

Sometimes when you have been in a position for a period of time, it is movement that makes you feel better, although the initial efforts are painful and stiff. As you now know, stiffness is an inference and a way of encouraging you to move to nourish your body. However, you can get caught up in a story that movement is 'dangerous' or possibly damaging and hence you avoid it. This is exactly the opposite of what we need and highlights the importance of understanding.

If your hand is painful, sometimes it is better to move other areas before to prime, change your state and willingness. Say it is your right hand. Initially, you can move your left hand: open and close your fingers, bend your wrist. Then extend and bend your left elbow, reach up in the air above your head, turn your head and neck and then start down your right-hand side. Finally, you move your right hand, but if it is sensitive, this may be gradual and less than the other side. But, considering the circumstances, this is the best decision right now to build upon. One good or better experience leads to another. Plus you have created evidence that you can move your right hand. It may not be moving exactly how you need it to yet—the keyword is yet. Implying a future when your movements will be better, which they can be.

Language

The words we use to ourselves have an impact, much as they do when delivered to other people. Except it's a double whammy for us. We are already feeling bad, and then the language we use makes us feel worse. The opposite will also be true.

Elsewhere I have talked about battlefield language: a war, winning the war, fighting, and so on. This is a common parlance in society, but we now know that there are issues with this approach. In effect, it guides you down an unhelpful path in most cases. Think of a battlefield and what is happening. Does this bear any resemblance to how you want to be? Does it promote healing and well-being?

Some may consider healing language to be woo or fluffy. However, when you think about what you want to achieve, then you can choose the words that are best for self-encouragement and motivation or to self-soothe.

For example, if you are in pain, you can say to yourself, 'there is the discomfort'. If it is burning, you can say 'warmth'. If you have had a day that you are telling yourself has been awful. Add a swear word if you like—research suggests it helps with pain (Stephens et al., 2011). You could say to yourself: 'It has been a day with many difficult moments, but also other times when I have felt other things such as joy or pleasure or relief.' This can be tricky, but it is possible. You may be thinking, no, it was a terrible day full stop. Understandable, but which direction do you want to point yourself now?

Mindful practice, which helps us gain insight into our experiences, will reveal the true nature of things, including the fact that we feel many different ways throughout the day. As you build your ability to be present, notice your inner dialogue and realise that it is but one viewpoint, you realise that you can take another. This is skilful self-coaching.

Other people or animals

Being with a loved one, a friend, someone who inspires you or your pet can change your state. This is self-soothing by choosing this action. A hug can feel great or just an understanding conversation—being listened to. In some cases, just being together in silence. Stroking a cat or dog will change your state as you bond with your pet.

Listening to a calm voice on a meditation app or a video has a strong effect on your autonomic nervous system. You don't have to actually be with that person.

Combinations

You may feel soothed soon after using one of these practices. Or it may take some time, but you have sowed the seeds. You also know about impermanence. In that sense, everything is short term because your state is constantly changing by the nature of living.

One action starts to apply the brakes, slow things down for you. Then you may add another in the space you have created. For example, breathing is a way to be present, which allows you to address your suffering. Then you decide to move. In time you will find out what works best for you, bearing in mind that what works now will most likely need updating at some point. Being curious about how things are for you helps. Cultivating an interest in how you experience things is another effect of regular mindful practice.

Your ways

You will already have some ways of self-soothing. If they work for you, great! Continue with these together with some of those mentioned above. It is about you and practices being helpful for you.

There are other skills you can practise such as RAIN and labelling (see Challenging moments), both ways of meeting the different situations you face moment to moment. Essentially, you are seeking to respond more and more skilfully, by seeing things for what they are, being in touch with reality and then creating the best conditions to move forward.

Encouragement points

- Self-soothing is an important skill that you will develop with practice.
- If you practise or rehearse at calm times, you will find it easier and more natural to apply when you need to.
- Self-soothing is about changing state in a direction where you feel better.
- Sometimes this happens quickly, other times you have to keep practising—sowing seeds.
- You will already have ways to self-soothe. What other ways can you add?

Breathing

'You are breathing, but are you breathing well? Your breath is one of the most accessible and powerful ways of changing state.' RS

To breathe is to be alive. Most of the time you breathe without thinking. When you become conscious of breathing, it often changes, just like walking. For some people, it is very difficult to breathe easily. Nonetheless, we are all breathing in our own way. This may or may not be efficient, having a significant impact on your health and sense of well-being.

It seems that many people do not breathe well. For a range of reasons, mouth breathing is common, despite the nose being the well-designed instrument it is for the respiration process. You may like to take a few moments to realise how you breathe. Nose or mouth? A combination perhaps. What happens when you walk? Faster? Upstairs? Ideally, you use your nose for both in and out.

People learning to breathe more effectively report feeling more energised, healthier, and better in themselves. There is also a calming effect that can be deeply relaxing. This is of great benefit, especially if life is full of challenges and hence stress (see Managing stress). Not only persistent pain is stressful because of the experience itself, but also the effects upon how you feel and the impact on your life (limitations, avoidances, etc.).

Much has been written on breathing and breathing practices. This section is not a comprehensive review, but rather an introduction together with some suggested exercises you can try. These are skills that I commonly teach people I see, and the ones that are most helpful. If you have any concerns about breathing exercises, please do consult with your healthcare profession.

Before I describe the practices, it is useful to have some understanding of why you would spend time doing this each day. There are many reasons why breathing skills are useful, including the following:

1. To be present
2. To create calm and clarity
3. To relax
4. To pause
5. To activate the parasympathetic nervous system
6. To improve your physiology
7. To manage difficult moments
8. To connect with your body
9. To help sleep
10. To ease pain

In addition to these clear benefits, you are also practising mindfulness and training yourself to pay attention. Being able to pay attention is well thought to be a skill of being well (Killington & Gilbert, 2010). This skill pervades out into other areas of your life as you improve your ability to be present, to see things as they are rather than the distortions of the mind.

Most of your biology is not under your direct control. Instead, it just happens. Your brain is managing your energy budget (Feldman-Barrett, 2021), anticipating what you may do next and allocating resources accordingly. There is nothing you need to do to increase your blood pressure to heart rate. There is nothing you can do; no button to push. You don't choose when you need to go to the toilet or when you feel hungry. Breathing is different. You can choose to change your breathing pattern or to observe the movements and other perceptions.

The effects that you will feel the most are those as a result of the parasympathetic nervous system (PSNS) becoming more active. As this happens, the sympathetic nervous system (SNS) (fight, flight, freeze) eases up. Together they constitute the autonomic nervous system (ANS), which is responsible for all the physiology that automatically keeps you alive. Important stuff then!

This in mind, having a way to positively influence the workings of these systems is a great asset.

The set up

Decide the length and style of your practice. Initially, this is a conscious decision, but with time you will notice how the habit forms and you will organically select without much or any effort.

When you start out, finding a comfortable position helps you to focus. I encourage sitting so that you are also alert; upright and relaxed are the words I often use. However, for some people, lying down is better. The risk is to fall asleep, which can be nice, but is not practice.

Place your hands where they feel most natural. Then gently close your eyes if you are comfortable to do so (some people don't like to).

The practices

Breathing awareness

This is the practice most often suggested by Thich Nhat Hanh, featuring in many of his talks and writings. Much of this work can be accessed on the Plum Village app.

You simply notice your breath as you breathe in and breathe out. Initially, this can be awareness of your chest and tummy expanding and then relaxing. Importantly, you do not try to control your breathing. You let it be—deep, shallow, short, long, whatever. With your full focus on your breath, you will notice the natural changes in pattern, seemingly without you doing anything at all. Less is more! As well as becoming aware of your breathing, you can also notice how you feel. You are the observer.

Once you have become aware of the movements of your body in relation to breathing, you can then zoom in to notice the feelings at the end of your nose. You are sharpening your focus.

It is very likely that during the practice, your mind will wander. This is normal and fine. To return your attention to your breath can be considered a 'rep' as in when you exercise, or an opportunity to refocus and get better at doing so. Some people worry about this and believe the they are doing something wrong. You are not. Just start again and keep going. Consistency in practice is key, even if it is just for a few moments.

You can add a mantra to help focus. For example:

- Breathing in, I am aware I am breathing in.
- Breathing out, I am aware I am breathing out.

Then, you can shorten it to: breathing in, breathing out.

Mantras can be created to be more specific. For instance, if you have noticed pain in your body:

- Breathing in, I know that a painful feeling is in there.
- breathing out, I calm that painful feeling.

At the end of your session, take a moment to notice how you feel, however that is. Try not to look for something or expect to feel a certain way. Acceptance of how things are right now is important and a skill in itself (see Acceptance). The opposite is resistance, which causes more suffering.

Mindful practices have become very popular. There are many books and apps available, promising a range of life-changing benefits. Yet the practice of mindfulness is not about getting anywhere and certainly not about relaxing or easing pain. However, these are the kinds of things that can happen when you practise consistently, but not by directly trying! Sounds paradoxical, I know.

I am hoping that you are starting to pick up on one of the main themes when overcoming pain, which links with what I have just said. Firstly, that consistency is key, but secondly that to feel better, unfortunately there is no button to press. Instead, you create the conditions for a better future by what you do right now. You cannot simply relax. What you can do is use breathing to create the conditions for a state of relation to emerge. It is the same with pain relief.

You cannot summon pain relief now if you are in pain because it is already happening. What you can do is to choose an action or sequence of actions that create the conditions for future relief—hopefully in the coming moments. Sometimes it takes more time, but if you can closely observe the ever-changing raw sensations and different feelings in your body, you will be in touch with what is really happening rather than getting caught up in the stories about what is happening. This allows you to ride the ups and downs, and respond with calm and clarity.

In the Mindfulness section I will go into more detail as to how you can become more observant of the raw sensations, seeing the difference between these and the stories (thoughts—mostly automatic) you tell yourself about what is happening. It is not so much what is happening that matters as much as how you relate to it. Is this thought true? Is it helpful?

How you relate to a situation makes it the way it is for you. As you know now, the way you relate and respond to a painful moment is something you can control. Learning to think about pain in line with modern science and philosophy helps relate in a resourceful way, leading to a best decision in that moment. Most of the suffering comes from the way you think about situations. Before you give it a meaning based on your existing beliefs, reactions, and preferences, it is a set of circumstances. Circumstances themselves have no feel until we relate to them in a particular way.

To do this you need to be present and able to see clearly, both skills that emerge from meditation and mindfulness practice.

Counting

There are different counting practices you can try. Here are some examples.

Once you have set up, you can start by noticing your body. After a few seconds or minutes, you can bring your attention to your breathing as it is.

a. 4/4: on connecting with your breath, you can count to 4 as you breathe in, and to 4 as you breathe out. If you find this too difficult, you can change the number. At the start, it is about establishing a rhythm, settling on a counting and breathing combination that feels comfortable.

   After some practice, you will find that the 4/4 pattern becomes easier. You can then progress to 5/5 and 6/6. Naturally this slows your breathing down.

b. The box: count to 4 as you breathe in, then hold your breath for 4, breathe out for 4 and hold for 4. This is the method apparently preferred by special forces to create calm and focus, which is understandable. You can also benefit as is the case with many practices that the elites and peak performers use.

When and how often to practise?

You are building a new habit, which means a consistent practice each day, like cleaning your teeth. Deciding the time you will practise can help groove the habit if you do it the same time day after day, until it becomes part of your normal routine. This always sounds easy.

There are a couple of principles to follow that can help. Firstly, set the bar low.

How many times a day will I definitely practise? The important word is definitely. There is also a feel to this; either of certainty, or uncertainty. This gives you a clue. The number you come up with does not matter as much as the fact that you have started. As I often say, one rep is better than none, and from there you will build.

You also need to decide how long you will practise. Again the question to self: how long will I definitely practise? 1 minute? 5 minutes? 10?

Now you have your target or baseline as a starter.

Say you have begun with 5 minutes, once a day. This is what you will definitely do as a minimum each day. You can do more of course, but always this.

Beyond your daily practice, there are also what I call micro-practices. This is when you take a few moments to yourself; a pause if you like. You could take one now.

Place the book down, adjust your position, close your eyes and follow 3 breaths in and out without trying to breathe any particular way. You are just aware of your breathing. That's it.

How was that?

To bring micro-practices into your day at regular points is a simple way to bring calmness and presence into your life. It will also have a positive effect on your energy levels. Some people find that a reminder or notification helps. I often suggest the bell of mindfulness on the Plum Village app (see Resources), which you can set to chime. It is a pleasant sound that you can come to associate with pausing and taking a moment for yourself. The clarity that comes gives you the space to notice what you might need and to make your next best decision.

So, in summary, there are two ways you can use a breathing practice:

1. Daily breathing awareness practice
2. Micro-practices through the day

When you have practised, acknowledge your win. Make it newsworthy and jot it down in your journal as a success if you like. It is easy to gloss over many achievements because they appear to you as being minor. This is only because there is a part of you that is critical or sets your expectations too high, as opposed to seeing what you have done as useful and another step in the right direction.

Together with noting your success, you can also reflect on the actual experience. What was it like for you? How did it feel and how do you feel now? This makes it whole inasmuch as you experience the embodiment of the thoughts and feelings rather than just thinking; the so-called living in your head. To increasingly notice how you embody thoughts and feelings is to connect with your body, a key part of being healthy and well.

Further, you can stack your new breathing habit upon something that you already do. For example, you may practise your breathing awareness once you have had a coffee. These two activities become linked so that one naturally leads to the other.

Remembering that this is a process rather than an end point helps you to see that one step leads to the next. You build a strong foundation by repeatedly practising at a low level and then gradually increase, if you want. It is your choice, weighing up the pluses and minuses.

When your mind wanders

This is inevitable. The human mind wanders. But as you practise, you will become more focused and present.

Some people feel that they must be doing it wrong if their attention moves around. No, you are doing your best.

In fact, when you notice that your mind has wandered, this becomes an opportunity to refocus. And again. And again. Like the repetition of an exercise such as a bicep curl. Through repetition you improve.

You cannot stop your mind wandering just as you cannot stop the tide coming in. But you can become more skilful at noticing when you do drift, and bringing your attention back to the object, in this case your breathing.

Breathing is happening all the time, largely without our awareness. Those suffering respiratory conditions such as COPD or asthma, together with people who regularly experience anxiety tend to notice the sensations of breathing more often because of their intensity and impact—shortness of breath and tightness are compelling, and readily grab attention. Learning to breathe better will have many benefits: for example, better oxygenation of the body and brain, calmness, increased energy. Also, knowing that you can use breathing more skilfully to create focus and calm gives a certain confidence.

Breathing and pain

In terms of pain, many people find that breathing techniques are an important part of getting better. Short, regular practices are proactive, build future health, and can often help during challenging moments.

Depending on the nature and intensity of the pain, breathing is a tool that you can use. From practising for a short time, many people find that breathing is effective in bringing some calmness, soothing and relief for low to moderately intense pain. If the pain is severe, breathing as a practice may not occur as essentially you are just trying to get through that moment however you can—perhaps even just surviving until you pass the peak, which you will.

If you deepen your practice over time, you will find that you can draw upon this skill at times when the feelings are more intense.

As with any positive action you take, there can sometimes be a quick change in state and experience of pain. At other times it may take longer. It is important to try and remember that if the pain does not change immediately, it does not mean that you are doing something wrong or that it does not work. There is always a time factor, which varies enormously according to many variables. And there are so many variables, at all times. The multitude of chemicals, nerves, signals, immune cells, and other factors at play in any given moment is unfathomable. Most of this you are unaware of as it is your biology in the dark.

So, what are you doing? You are creating the conditions for a calmer state to emerge in time. Pain relief is always in the future, not now. If you are in pain now, you are in pain now. That moment has emerged in service of what has come before, which is the same for the coming moments.

Pain being such a compelling experience, we want relief now. Realising the true nature of things means we can set our expectations according to what is rather than what is not. This may sound a little philosophical. Perhaps it is, but this is an important point that makes a huge difference. Becoming lost in the thoughts that you want relief now, and nothing else will do, whilst understandable, only puts all your energy and focus onto your pain and suffering. This is when things feel worse, by focusing on what you don't want (pain) rather than what you do (feel better).

In time and with practice, including breathing, we can become aware of our responses and shape them more skilfully as we direct our actions towards a future that features increasing wellness, pleasure, and joy.

Using breathing to achieve success

I would like to share with you a couple of ways that we use breathing in sessions to help with moving and dealing with feeling pain. Remember that one of the main principles for getting better is to have better experiences. You create situations (experiments) and curate them to be such, setting yourself up for a likely win that you can build upon.

1. Priming (also see section on Priming)

Priming is what you can do to get into the best state for something you are about to do, and hence get the best result that you can, always considering the circumstances. Common examples that we see are the way athletes prepare before an event (imagery, self-talk, certain movements—watch Steve Smith the Australian cricketer go through his routine before each ball) or a singer using vocal exercises prior to the performance. You could think of it as getting into the right mindset or perhaps mood, so that you can focus on what you are doing.

Breathing is a way to prime. Firstly, you can check in and notice how you are in the present moment.

'How am I?' is a useful question to start. You can scan your attention through your body, becoming aware of any tension or discomfort, which if not addressed will be carried into the next task. Think of the person who has been sitting at their desk all day, not moving very often, who decides to go for a run. Without checking in, noticing stiffness and tension, they will take that stiff, tense body into the run. This increases the risk of pain and injury versus consciously easing that tension and stiffness with movement and breathing before then running with a more pliable body.

I think it is worthwhile remembering at this point that we are a whole. In other words, there is no actual separation of mind and body. You are a whole person who has a single lived experience of what it is like to be you. The way you think and feel and perceive the world around you is grounded in the state of your body. Equally, your body state informs the way you think and feel. It all comes together; embodied.

The practice of breathing awareness brings you to the present moment enables you to deal with whatever needs your attention before starting the intended activity. This maybe a few breaths or longer if you feel the need for a deeper practice. You can also combine breathing with imagery or movement as a way of priming for a particular action.

2. Sitting with your pain

When I write or say sitting with your pain, there is actually sitting with your pain. It is also a metaphor for something you can learn to do when pain is your experience in that moment, while you are in a particular situation or doing something.

Firstly, literally sitting with your pain. You could also be lying down.

Bring your attention to your body, noticing all and any feelings as they arise (and pass). What is it like to be sitting as you are? Next, pay gentle attention to your breathing: the movement, the air flowing in and out of your nose.

After a few moments, move your attention, like a spotlight, to an area of pain or discomfort. Notice what happens when you put your attention on your pain—attention works like a volume switch. Now you can examine your pain experience and see what happens as time passes by. You may start to get the sense that it is dynamic and changing (it is but we don't always realise) moment by moment; the qualities, the intensity, the thoughts about it.

Whilst paying attention to your pain, you continue to breathe in an easy, gentle way, maintaining that parasympathetic state as best you can. This is a skill of course, which means you will get better in time.

As you sit and breathe, opening your awareness to your pain, you are learning to be with and to transform the experience. As with any transformation to make things better, we must turn and face the suffering. This requires courage but also compassion. This can be a difficult exercise, and sometimes it can feel impossible. That's ok. You can choose to do something else, or nothing at all. This is the compassion and self-caring bit that matters.

When you don't do something or have been able to achieve a certain level, a part of you may be critical or unkind. Knowing and hearing that part of you with another part of you that is caring and patient, can really help with the healing process (see Compassion).

To start, you may practise sitting and breathing awareness for just a few moments. As with moving, you are trying to create good experiences that you can build on. A good experience is one where on balance you feel that you have learned something useful and taken a step (sometimes small, but a step nonetheless) in the right direction. There may well have been some pain, but within your window of tolerance.

In this practice you are crafting better and more skilful responses to your pain, feeling more control bit by bit.

Similar to sitting with your pain to transform the experience, you can apply this to a chosen activity or movement. We can use bending as an example, a movement that is often feared or avoided by people suffering back pain.

As an aside, there are many messages 'out there' about bending when you have back pain. There are similar messages for bending to pick things up, pointing out the potential risk for back injuries if you don't use your legs. This may be seen in a different light when you understand that the most important movement for a healthy back is to bend. We need bending!

Initially you can check in as described above. Then bring your attention to your breathing (easy, gentle rhythm). Think about the movement you are going to make, and then begin whilst continuing to breathe. Some people like to time their breath and movement.

For instance, as you breathe in, reach and bend within your window of tolerance, and then as you breathe out, come back up. Moving like this creates evidence that it is safe to move, enhanced by the calmness of breathing smoothly. Repeated episodes start to shift the expectation and prediction of pain towards that of moving more freely and confidently.

What role does breathing play? It keeps you present, focused, aware and as Thich Nhat Hanh says, it brings you home.

Encouragement points

- Learning to breathe well is a skill that builds wellness through the biological effects; for example, better oxygenation of your body and brain.
- Breathing is a way to practice being present. This is the only time that you can self-care.
- Breathing is a way to create calm and clarity, easing overwhelming feelings and suffering—applying the brakes.
- Regular practice helps you develop your skill and to be able to move into a better state.
- The breath is something you can be aware of as a practice, or a way to initiate more parasympathetic (restorative, healing, anti-inflammatory) activity.

Touch

'We have a whole system dedicated to soothing and loving touch to access.' RS

There is perhaps nothing more human than touch when it comes to caring for someone. A hand on the back or shoulder, to take another's hand, or to gently stroke are all acts that comfort and demonstrate presence and concern.

Touch is one of the senses that requires an object—something or someone to touch. Metaphorically though, you can also touch another person's heart or wider still, a nation can be touched by the acts of an individual. For example, many people have been touched by the compassion and life work of Thich Nhat Hanh who recently passed away. Also known as Thay, meaning teacher, he spoke instead of his death, of his continuation in the way that we live.

Maybe there is someone you have been touched by in this way. Perhaps you know them or have just read their words. Either way, they have had a positive influence on you, the way you think and live. If you have, and I hope you have, take a moment to picture them and notice how you feel. This is a practical way of being in touch, taking advantage of the fact that interbeing is truth. It was Thich Nhat Hanh who came up with this term to describe how we are connected together rather than separate as individuals.

Touch with your hands has a different quality and there are various experiences you can have. When you touch an object, you feel the quality of that object. If you pick up your phone, there can be a sense of its shape and size determined by how you have to position your hand and the way you use your fingers to grip it. You may feel a coolness, a hardness, but also some pleasure if you are attached to your phone—some people love the feel of it.

Compare this to being asked to put your hand through a hole into a box without knowing what is contained within. As you reach in, you feel something cold, wet, and slimy. Notice that the descriptions you use don't tell you about the object itself. You need confirmation from vision.

You may have realised that touch and vision have objects: you touch something or you see something. With pain, there is no object, making it a unique experience. I can touch and see my leg, but I can't 'pain' something. Realising this truth helps us to understand our pain not only as a perception, but what it is actually like. In this, we can come to know how it changes according to the present circumstances.

Touch is understood to be the first sense we develop in the womb (Gottlieb, 1976). Then it plays a significant role in healthy emotional development and of our sense of self (Ciaunica et al., 2021) (this is me and that is the world—although there may not be the separation that is first thought; see 'What is pain?' section to understand the enactive viewpoint). Imagine a world without touch or the inability to feel, as some must endure.

Dr Paul Brand's book The Gift of Pain, co-authored with Philip Yancey (1997) documents his work as a doctor in India working with people suffering the effects of leprosy. He discovered that their inability to feel pain caused the injuries and subsequent infections, disfigurements, amputations, and hence suffering. Similar to those few who are congenitally insensitive to pain (CIP), lifespan is shortened because the person has no way of knowing that there is an injury or that their body integrity is threatened.

Imagine a small stone in your shoe. How irritating and painful this can be as you walk along and its sharp edge presses into the sole of your foot. The touch of the stone, indenting the skin. You notice it because your brain predicts that the sharp feeling is the best explanation for the experience, based on past events. You stop, adopt that awkward one-legged posture as you remove your shoe, shake it out, and try to see the guilty stone fall onto the floor. On putting your shoe back on, you can resume walking as normal.

Now imagine you did not have the ability to detect that sharp stone in your shoe. You keep walking and it gradually breaks the skin. Inflammation and healing kick in. But it is warm and sweaty in your shoe, creating a superb environment for bacteria that can now enter the wound. You can see where this may go if the person does not know that this is happening. If they do not visibly check their feet, how would they know? One of the simple practices that Brand encouraged, or rather, insisted upon, was that the people he cared for must regularly check their feet. Much like diabetics who have neuropathy with altered sensation.

Recent times with lockdown due to COVID-19 resulted in many people being starved of touch. Even when opportunities to touch normally offered themselves, such as a handshake or a hug, they would be avoided just in case. Kissing loved ones became a source of consideration, a risk analysis, rather than a connection. Fortunately, it seems we are moving on and touch has become more thoughtless and effortless once more.

Professor Frances McGlone from Liverpool University has been investigating touch for many years. He didn't mince his words when he spoke about the importance of touch: 'Touch isn't just good—it's absolutely essential. Denying it is like denying a child oxygen. I get very exercised about the demonisation of touch. It's cruel, in my mind. It's another form of abuse.' His work has revealed much about the biology of touch and the nerves that preferentially respond to light touch, the CT fibres (C tactile). More on this below.

Touch and pain

Both touching the world and being touched can become an unpleasant experience in pain. Now there is another layer within the quality of what it is like, and one that can be anticipated fearfully or at least expected. Unfortunately, thinking that something will hurt beforehand can make it more likely that it will, and more. This kind of expectation resides subconsciously as well as being an overt thought. Sometimes you may not be thinking that a movement or action will hurt, but then it does.

Pain intrudes and becomes consuming, defining and filling the moment instead of thoughtless and effortless movement. Normally we know that we have a body, as this is how we are in the world, but it does not obscure what we are doing. Pain becomes a crack in the window. Instead of seeing a glassless view, you see the split close up.

Of course, you are not going looking for the pain. It is simply part of your perception of the world, your world, unbidden and certainly not chosen, yet definitely there. Like all perceptions, pain appears as the content of your consciousness. There is nothing that you need to do for it to arise, much like sounds, smells, and what you see. In that circumstance, they are just present.

The objects that you touch or pick up can feel substantially different. For instance, you may grasp something soft, yet it feels sharp or hard. Then there is the difference because of the pain itself, which you may or may not have been expecting. It can seem strange, peculiar, or even disturbing. Once you understand that our perceptions are being generated as predictions about the object rather than the object itself, it can start to make sense.

Another common perception is the size of the body or body part. Not related to touch particularly, I think it is important to mention. These less usual or downright bizarre feelings can be scary, and even sound odd when you describe them to yourself. Consequently, many people keep these changes in bodily experiences to themselves for fear of not being believed.

There can already be an issue with being taken seriously because you cannot see pain (you can never see the pain but people seem to forget that point) and hence point to show someone. People are still disbelieved—unbelievably in 2023—adding to the misery. There is something more real about things that can be seen in some people's eyes, which is clearly wrong thinking.

The more often you touch and feel pain together, in a way the more likely it will keep happening, unless you can create other evidence to suggest a different experience. This is the basis of getting better as you know. Creating and curating such experiences that you can gradually build upon and progress at the right time.

To be touched and it hurt has a different kind of quality. The pain can still intrude and most certainly transforms a caress into a source of suffering rather than pleasurable. This would be the case with allodynia, which is the experience of pain in circumstances when you would not expect it: light touch is painful, often agonising. The predicted state is one of pain despite the context being normal, loving touch, or the light contact of a sleeve, the bedcovers, or even a cool draft. When it comes to intimacy, this is the most troubling of pains.

Now, despite these changes, there are ways that you can use touch to be soothed and to self-soothe. This is one way that someone else can help you, when other people often do not know what they can do. For partners it can be worrying as they fear hurting you, but equally want to touch and be close. Below are some practical ways that touch can be used effectively, starting with how you can be touched by another person. Perhaps you hand the book to them, or you read it together.

But just before the practice, here is some important background.

We have a system dedicated to gentle touch that is for bonding and soothing. It is there, ready to predict the experience of pleasure but is considered to have a prosocial role in bonding—we have a system dedicated to togetherness and connection.

Think about how you would touch someone who is suffering. It would most likely be a gentle hand on the shoulder or back, and then perhaps a slow caress as you brush your hand over their body. You may accompany this with a particular voice tone that is comforting. In one way you are slowing everything down: what you say, what you do and in so doing, create the conditions for calmness.

Another way to think about this is the caring a parent gives to a baby or your child. The gentle stroking of the skin to help them fall asleep or to soothe them if they have fallen or feel unwell. The action of gentle stroking stimulates particular nerve endings that are dedicated to this kind of touch—CT fibres (or C tactile). Studies have shown that stroking 1–10 cm per second is the optimal speed, which turns out to be the loving touch or caring concern style of touch (Loken et al., 2009).

You know that they have been activated because the feeling is pleasurable rather than something else. These nerves also respond to temperature, so having a warm hand helps (Ackerley et al., 2014). You probably know what it is like when someone puts a cold hand on your back! It's the opposite of this.

Paying attention to how you stroke is important. When I teach people how to stroke, I also describe it as like stroking a cat, to give you the sense of what you are doing. There is a tendency to go with the hairs as well: from the elbow to the hand, for example, as it is mainly hairy skin where the CT fibres are found. The experiments show that the stroking needs to be:

Soothing touch: To another

There are three ways (at least) that you can soothe, show caring concern, and actually create the conditions for pain relief via the medium of touch as a partner, parent, or friend.

1. *Light stroking*

With a warm hand (normal skin temperature), you stroke the area, working with the other person to make sure that it feels pleasant. You may have to adjust the speed and the lightness of your pressure.

If the area is too sensitive, then you can work outside it, perhaps just touching the boundary. In time, you will be able to move closer and into the sensitive zone. You can also stroke the other side to gain the mirror effect. Once you have stroked the other side, you can move across. The area that is sensitive can change from day to day, and sometimes moment to moment—it is dynamic.

I suggest that the stroking continue for at least 30–40 reps, but if it feels good, you can continue.

Afterwards, you can move the area to nourish. Often, if a movement is difficult because of stiffness or pain (or both), it becomes easier to practise and hence a good experience to build upon. Hopefully you can see how this, and the other forms of touch described below can become part of your day-to-day practice.

2. *Holding hands*

It has been shown that when partners hold hands, there is a pain-relieving effect (Goldstein et al., 2018). What a simple thing to do!

3. *Mild pressure massage*

The amount of pressure you apply is enough that it can be felt by the recipient, but not so much that there is any tensing up. In most cases, it should feel pleasant. At this level, a parasympathetic response will be evoked (Diego & Field, 2009), which is felt as relaxing and calming.

The parasympathetic nervous system is a branch of the autonomic system, responsible for coordinating restorative processes. It works together with the SNS that you may have heard of as 'flight or fight'. There is also a third lesser-known element: freeze. This system mobilises resources when there is a possible or actual danger. One of the most common feelings associated with this system is anxiety, which interestingly, feels very similar to excitement.

Notice that this is a great example of context and the story. Both of these make a situation what it really is for you. If you are feeling a particular way and you call it anxiety, what happens if you change your story to excitement?

Similar to stroking, your partner can apply the mild pressure massage on areas away from the sensitive zone and gradually work inwards within a session or over time. For pure relaxation, if this is a practice for you, then having a regular massage to ease tense parts of your body can be helpful.

By exploring and connecting with your body in this way, you can discover how you respond to different areas receiving this attention. As you know now, connecting (or reconnecting) with your body is an important part of healing and getting better. By staying present during the treatment and following the feelings of touch, you can deepen your sense of connection and notice pleasant perceptions of touch and your body.

Having endured pain for some time, this becomes the predominant experience and expectation for many people. With this kind of practice, and the others (notice that this is a theme: creating evidence for getting better and having good experiences of your body), you are purposely creating and noticing bodily sensations with an overall feeling of pleasure and calmness. This is newsworthy and great material for your journal of wins.

Following the treatment, you can practise movements to make it part of a useful sequence. Or sometimes you may practise breathing or something else that maintains a calm and present state.

Soothing touch: To self

You can also apply these techniques to yourself. Of course, it is not quite the same and indeed there are different patterns of neural activity in the brain and spinal cord (Boehme et al., 2019). It can be hard to tell the difference between being touched and being the toucher.

Nonetheless, there is an effect of using touch that can be useful for soothing but also as a primer before you practise a movement. Commonly after a period of stroking (e.g. 30–40 strokes) and connecting positively with your body, movement quality and range improves. Essentially you have changed state by using touch—the same applies to all the touch-based practices mentioned here. In this change, you are able to move better and build your repertoire.

Some people find that when they are stroking, looking at the area helps as well. This can be done directly by turning your head or by watching in a mirror. See which works best for you.

Encouragement points

- Touch is a very human way of connecting and bending with others and ourselves.
- Touch can be pain relieving, soothing, and used as a practice.
- We have a specialised system of nerve endings for gentle touch, dedicated to affiliation, soothing, and bonding.
- Different types of touch can be used to induce calmer and better states.
- Touch is one way that others can be helpful.

Movement

'Movement is fundamental for healthy living, nourishing the whole of you. When you know how, the world starts to look like a different place.' RS

There is not a lot you can achieve without movement. It is fundamental for living, influences how the world appears to you, your opportunities for action and to maintain the health of your body and brain.

Of course, movement can hurt. Sometimes it is expected such as after a new workout in the gym or an unaccustomed long walk. This is part of the way that the body is adapting to what you have done. It may be very uncomfortable, yet this is normal. When you can explain it away to yourself, whilst the pain and soreness still exists, your suffering is minimised. You also know that it will come to an end soon—it is not permanent.

Normally movement happens without much or any thought. It is effortless in that way, although it can be hard work. Your body is transparent, meaning that you know it is there but not intruding on your ability to move. You have confidence in what you are about to do, knowing you can rely on your body to move as you wish, most of the time. Occasionally you may mis-step, bump into something, or knock something over.

Movement is a different experience when you suffer chronic pain. The body is very present and becomes a source of doubt (Carel, 2008). 'I can' becomes 'can I'? Or 'how can I'? Or 'I can't'. There is another layer plus scrutiny of the environment and anticipation that certain movements or positions will be painful. This consumes a lot of energy. The world appears in a very different way when suffering chronic pain, literally. As you will see, the way we move is playing a role in generating your experience of being you and the environment in which you find yourself.

Learning how to move better includes feeling safe, building confidence, developing body sense for economy and precision of movement and gradually moving focus away from the body and fearful thoughts to just doing. You need movement to do things in your environment but movement also nourishes your body and brain. It is muscular contraction and relaxation that pumps blood and oxygen round your body together with the heart.

There is overwhelming evidence of the benefits of movement, activity, and exercise on long-term health. It is the magic pill. Clearly you need movement to pursue your purpose, another key factor for health and well-being. In fact, all the skills of well-being require some kind of movement. But you need to know how to do it.

When you move, you are fulfilling a prediction that the brain and other body systems (e.g. immune, endocrine; tying together how you feel, general health, ability to move, think, and perceptions of the world) have already made. If the movement or activity was painful before, the brain can predict that this time it is painful as well, even if there is no real danger or threat to your integrity. Some people feel pain even before they have moved in anticipation or when they watch someone else move in a way that they expect would hurt. This can be very confusing. But we can explain this now by understanding the brain as a predictor, not a responder.

With movement being so important for your health and to live well, you have to find ways of building confidence and reducing sensitivity. Fortunately, there are a number of ways, starting with understanding what is happening and why it hurts when you do simple things. Deepening your knowledge of your experiences and why you have them helps reduce worry and distress. Both further activate the threat system and hence can increase the chance of feeling pain. Starting to feel safe to move is a significant step forward. In this state, you can practise movements and activities to create evidence that you are doing well instead of the opposite.

Action, thinking, and perception

In addition to understanding pain (see section What is pain?), it is useful to have some insights into perception—your conscious experience. This is your reality and it is being generated by your body systems. This is your version of events if you like.

Whilst there is a world out there and you have a body, you are creating the experience of what it is like; that is, your perception. This is being shaped by many things. Your expectations, past experiences, beliefs, attention, mood, and emotions are all playing a role. This is why your perceptions are unique to you and changeable. This gives great hope when it comes to pain, which can feel like it won't change, or sometimes you are actually told that it won't change. Many people have been told that this is how it will be and now you have to manage or cope. This is just not true. Things are changing all the time. Life would not be possible otherwise, which in turn opens up possibilities for you to get better.

The lived experience, or what it is like to be you right now (there is only this moment that is real, the rest is imagined—future and past are not happening), sits at the centre of what you think, perceive, and are doing. There is no separation of these factors. Similarly, there is no actual separation of mind and body. This is only in your thinking. Reality is a unified experience. You are a whole person with a continuously changing experience.

Experience, contemplation, and science tell us that action, perception, and thought come together, meaning that they influence each other. We think by the fact that we have our body and a brain that work together. Our actions are shaped by our thoughts, mood, and perceptions. Our perceptions are being created through our thinking and actions.

Some simple examples help illustrate the point. Out loud, pretend that you are giving directions to a friend, how to get from the station to your house. Notice what you do with your body.

Now repeat the exercise, but sit on your hands. Also, don't move your head or eyes. What is the difference?

When you are tired, the stairs look steeper. If you are standing on the top of a hill on a skateboard, it will look different to someone standing on the ground.

When you suffer chronic pain, things can look further away (Witt et al., 2009).

As you know now, you are generating this experience. It is not the outside world in, it is inside out, top down. Each person has their own perception of any given situation based on all their learnings and experiences to date. If you watch a film with someone or look at a painting together, you will have a different experience. There may be some things you agree on, but colours, for example, are unique to you. Colour is not out there in the world. Instead, you create the colour. Green, you both say. But how do you know what kind of green the other person is seeing?

Importantly, this individual generation of experiences creates opportunities to shape a positive future by building healthy habits, learning to self-care, be skilful with your inner dialogue, and improve your mobility and movement, amongst other things.

Now let's apply this knowledge from enactivism and embodied cognition to movement. The essence of it is to have good experiences that you can build upon. To get better, you need to create evidence that you can do things and feel better. This is achieved with your daily practices that you can think of as experiments but also within day-to-day activities: how can I make this a good experience? Firstly, you work within your window of tolerance by thinking about what you can do. Taking breaks and making sure that your expectations and reality are aligned. Finally, acknowledging your success logs the win, remembering that each time you have a good experience it becomes the prior for next time. These are all covered elsewhere in the book.

Motion is lotion

This is a term that I use to help people understand the benefits of moving. All of our tissues (muscles, tendons, nerves, bones, etc.) need movement to be healthy. They are nourished by regular motion, hence the idea of lotion. Sit still for a few hours on a long car journey or to watch a film. Then, on getting up, how does your body feel?

It is simple. We are designed to move. It is how we eat, survive, and procreate. Beyond the basic functions, we also like to play sports, visit museums, go for walks with the dog, look around, scratch our heads, and much more. Even when we talk many of us use movement beyond the mouth. Try giving directions whilst sitting on your hands for instance. Breathing, the essence of life …

Moving and making contact with the world gives us sensory information that the brain can predict the meaning of and hence create our perceptions.

Have you ever tried to write after lying on your arm when it goes numb? When the sense of your arm temporarily disappears? That body sense is being generated by your body systems, like all other experiences that appear in your awareness. When there is then a mismatch between what is (subconsciously) expected and the sense data that arrives, this creates an error that is felt as the body feels different. This is more common than you may expect with chronic pain—altered body sense. The expectation is to feel whole and fully intact, but the sensory information says something else because of a change in signalling. The nerves in your arm are sending different or fewer messages that do not match the prediction. This is newsworthy and can be felt as numbness or detachment.

Movement is an active way of minimising that error so that your arm feels like yours once more. In chronic pain, minimising the error may not happen so quickly and usually needs consistent training over a period of time to bring the expectations (predictions) and reality (sensory data) back in alignment. This is more specific sensorimotor training when you would also use other senses to get a better grip on what is actually happening.

When you move, your muscles contract and relax, pumping blood and oxygen through the body. The bigger the movements, the more you nourish.

For example, after typing for a while, you can fully extend your fingers and then make a fist, rotate your wrists, bend, and straighten your elbows, reach up with your hands, look left and right, and turn to look behind you. Typing involves many small and precise movements that send a lot of noise into the system. Getting a good grip on what is happening can be challenging at times, bringing a mismatch in expectation and reality that results in aches and pains (the errors). This is the scenario for upper limb problems associated with typing and keyboards (i.e. repetitive strain injury—when there is frequently no injury!).

Of course, it is not just about keyboards, chairs, and desk heights. It is about a thinking, feeling, living human being with a lifetime of experiences shaping the present moment.

Movement, then, is a healthy habit, to look after yourself and your body as well as a way to achieve goals and live life.

Many people spend a long time sitting. Gradually the tissues creep as the pressure is maintained over time. Blood and nutrients are pushed out of the tissues and the acid levels build up. That can be uncomfortable. The message is to move. Add sensitivity to the picture and quickly this can become painful.

'Motion is lotion' is a healthy habit. A way of having regular and consistent good experiences of movement.

Movement habits

You can build a movement practice into your day as a new healthy habit. There are particular times of the day when this can be useful. For instance, a routine in the morning can help ease stiffness and set the day up in a positive way.

Through the day you can choose different movements or exercises, and changes of position (e.g. sitting to standing, using a standing desk) to nourish and refresh both how your body feels and how you are generally. Thinking is clearer when your body feels better. You will make better decisions.

Essentially you can become the type of person who moves consistently in order to improve and sustainably maintain the health of your body tissues and hence you as a whole. If you are suffering from chronic pain, this will be step by step. Some people find that a reminder or prompt helps build consistency. For example, notes, sticky dots, or a phone notification. I like the Plum Village app that has the Mindful Bell, which can be set to chime as often as you wish to be reminded.

Each time you practise, this is another step towards the more active version of you, even if it is one rep or just a few moments. As I say to people I work with, one rep is always better than none.

Novel and practical movements

You move in many different ways. In a clinic examination you are often asked to bend forward, reach up, and turn that way. However, in reality you move in multiple directions at once. To reach up for something, you may have to lean your body and turn your head, or to put on your shoe, you need to stand on one leg, flex and rotate your hip, and bend forward.

There are many combinations and varieties depending on the state you are in, the context, and the aim of the movement. If you have been sitting for some time, you may be stiffer, meaning that bending and twisting is a little harder, more uncomfortable, and less mobile (than if you had been walking or moving).

As well as movements in one plane, combinations are important to include. Some of these you will have discovered because when you moved that way, it was painful or restricted. Often people then avoid those movements for fear of injury or the pain itself. This is understandable, but it means that the movement becomes even stiffer and more painful over time. What we actually need to do is to work within the window of tolerance and explore that movement. Organically then it can increase because you are having good and better experiences, reducing the perceived threat and nourishing the tissues.

The window of tolerance is when you work within a range that feels good or at least tolerable for you, in that moment. It also means that you can continue with what you need to do afterwards and don't have to retreat to the couch or bed or stop what you are doing except for a scheduled recharge break. This means you are creating a good or better experience of movement that can be built upon—good movements lead to more good movements. Why? Because previous experiences are shaping the current one.

When you have identified specific movements combinations or directions that are problematic, you can start making those movements bit by bit. If there is sensitivity or fear, you can use imagery as a primer. When you imagine making the movement, your brain is doing some similar things to when you actually move.

Creating good experiences of movement

Movement can be feared because of pain, mainly due to prior experiences that inform the present. This is both consciously (I think this will hurt because it has done so before and why would I think anything else?) and subconsciously (the brain using past experience to establish the best explanations for what is happening now). People know that moving and being active is important for health, but with this fear and a history of it hurting, it is understandable why someone would choose to limit their movements or avoid them. The problem with this is the downward spiral. The existing level of activity reduces and the associated fear or concern increases. Deconditioning is part of this as general fitness and tolerance for activity diminishes, making it harder and harder to do normal daily things: washing, dressing, walking, cleaning, and cooking.

So how can you turn this around? Well, you can, but just need a way. The first step is to understand your pain and what is happening. Many people tell me how much better they feel by simply understanding their pain. It is as if the door is unlocked. With the practical understanding of pain, re-engaging with movement and activity becomes easier—although not necessarily easy.

The aim is to curate a good experience. You set the parameters and the goal to maximise the chances of success. This is what you then build upon moving forward, gradually switching deeper expectations from the movement to be painful to something better and better. It is a step-by-step process, whereby you are bringing your own conscious expectations in line with the reality of the circumstances. There is a certain amount that you can do that would be within the window of tolerance. This is the level that you can tolerate, which does not evoke great concern or much impact at all, and you can continue with what you were doing afterwards. On reflection, you are able to look back and feel that you have been successful.

Acknowledging success is an important part of the practice. You are actively creating evidence of what you can do, which is a key part of getting unstuck. The stickiness appears to set in when we repeatedly do worse than expected over time. Initially we think that we will get better, but then we don't. In time, the way it looks starts to shift towards an expectation that things will just hurt—a painful world. Noticing the good stuff becomes increasingly difficult when we are stuck because this is not what we expect anymore. This is like a person who grows up in a difficult environment that causes stress. Both consciously and subconsciously, there is an expectation that this is how the world is, even when there is no actual stressor. The body's systems continue to anticipate, prepare for, and respond to stress because of what is known can happen. This continues until some other credible evidence emerges. That is what you are now seeking to create in the things you do.

You become a scientist, making an experiment. Deciding what you will do, how much, and when, you are creating an opportunity to succeed. When your expectations (set by the experiment) meet or exceed the reality, it feels good—an achievement. The bar has been set purposely low so that it increases the likelihood of success, and as I have said above, you can then build on this.

Expanding your choices and opportunities

Pain intervenes between you and the environment. Activities and movements you would normally do without thought and with an invisible body (you know it is there but without any intrusion or doubt) now require planning or even a decision as to whether you will engage or not.

For example, opening a door. You would typically take the handle and turn it to achieve your goal. Now you have hand pain. Notice how this intervenes. Do you try anyway? Do you use your other hand? What will be the cost?

Painful movements impact enormously on life, because for most things we need to move. Even scratching your head. The world appears differently when you are suffering pain. The choices and opportunities narrow, which is another cause of suffering as you are unable to live in the way you wish or need. The opposite is also true. By increasing your movement choices and repertoire, more opportunities are available to you within the environment.

Thinking of moving as a skill means you can consider practice to be an important part of getting better. And as with any practice, quality, repetition, and feedback are key to taking a step forward towards your picture of success.

Movement experiments

There may be movements that you fear, worry about, or avoid (if you can) because you think they will hurt. This expectation has become a higher belief, feeling somehow certain because of the times beforehand when it hurt. Now there is a choice. Is it helpful to continue avoidance or do you need to engage with that movement and bring it back into your repertoire?

Now there is an association of a particular movement and pain within a certain context or situation. It could be standing up from a chair, bending over, or reaching up. This cannot be unlearned per se but can be replaced gradually with better movement that feels easier. These are movement experiments (experiences) that you set up in order to maximise chances of success, and perhaps even do better than expected.

Initially, you create calm and clarity using breathing awareness to be present in a comfortable position. You can think of this as a particular state—biological and how you feel. Imagery and visualisation help to deepen the state. For instance, think of a loved one or a time when you have been successful.

Notice how your state changes as you put your focus on this, remembering that what we focus on governs how we feel. Further, before and during you can self-soothe and reassure with certain messages: for example, I am safe to move, my body needs movement, movement is healthy. You can do this because of your new understanding of pain.

The movement you choose to practise follows the principles that you know including remaining within your window of tolerance. This means that you may feel various things but on balance, low or no impact and you can continue afterwards as planned. There is no need to push at all. Having repeated good experiences will result in natural progression.

During the movement remain present as best you can, reminding yourself that you are safe and that your body needs this nourishment. You are aware of the difference between the state of your body tissues and your experience of your body moving—one is objective and one subjective. The number of repetitions has been set that is ideal.

Set the bar low so that you make it likely you will succeed. The main goal, however, is to have the intent and then actually practice. If you are working within your window of tolerance, you may take a break before the reps are completed. This flexibility is important. The fact that you have done some of them is what counts rather than forcing through, which often leads to unnecessary extra pain.

This is focusing on the process over the prize. In the long term, being present, consistent, and flexible, the prize will take care of itself.

Your mindful practice will be helping you as you examine your own experiences more closely and notice the variability, the dynamic nature of our feelings, and essentially the difference between what is really happening and what you are telling yourself about what is happening. The two can sit apart, yet the story often wins out. This means it is easy to believe that you are doing worse than you really are, when in fact there are times when you feel better or good. The latter is the evidence you need, hence the suggestion of logging daily wins (see Journal).

We are, of course, where possible, aiming to move towards thoughtless actions when we know we have a body, but it is to a large extent invisible. You are what you are doing in this case. When this is not possible, we can still aim to move in the best way, knowing that with ongoing practice, it will get better in time.

Encouragement points

- We need movement to achieve our goals.
- Movement is a skill that can be practised so that your opportunities and choices grow.
- Understanding your pain helps you re-engage with movement.
- Movement is one of the ways we build our health.
- You can create movement experiments so that you increase the likelihood of being successful and building on this success.
- Everything you do is a practice for the next time.

Morning routine

'There is something very positive about starting the day with a positive intent and few successes.' RS

There is something positive about starting the day with some success. A famous and well-watched speech on YouTube by Admiral William McRaven starts by suggesting you make your bed (see video on YouTube). He goes on to explain that this is a job done that leads to the next and the next. At the end of the day, you come back to that made bed, whatever has happened in the between hours.

Some people suffering from chronic pain find making the bed difficult or impossible. It is not something they can do, yet. However, there are many other tasks that can be performed successfully to get the day started.

Here is a simple routine that I suggest to people I see in the clinic. You can build on it in your own way of course.

Three steps:

Breathe

Spend a few minutes breathing in and out through your nose. Sitting upright and relaxed is best, but if you need to lie down, this is fine as well. Just try not to fall back to sleep!

Depending on the time you have, it may be just a few breaths to oxygenate the body and brain, or a few minutes to gain clarity and feel and sense of building energy.

Visualisation is also an option during the breathing practice. You may think about your favourite place or a loved one and note the feelings in your body.

Move

Once you have oxygenated your body and eased some of the tension by activating the parasympathetic nervous system, you can introduce some easy movement to nourish your body.

You can choose which areas you move. Sometimes moving easier areas first helps to change state so that the stiffer areas are then more comfortable to nourish.

Set out your intent for the day

What will be your style, approach, and attitude today?

Deciding what this will be forms an intent. You may also visualise yourself in this state. Again, feel this in your body.

Some people create a mantra that they repeat to themselves or choose three words that best decide that version of themselves. We can set a reminder on our phones of these words so that there is an opportunity to check in through the day.

We can work on this version and other versions of ourself as a practice. For example, the compassionate self. We clarify what this self looks like and how it is characterised accompanied by the feelings of what it is like. Then we step into those shoes.

Energy

> '*Managing your energy is like managing your bank account. When you spend, you also need to save.*' RS

How would you score your level of energy right now, out of 10? ___/10

On average, how would you score your level of energy over the past week, out of 10? ___/10

Answering these questions will give you an insight into how you are managing your energy day to day and moment to moment. To manage your energy is a skill.

We get energy from sleeping, eating well, pursuing a purpose, exercising, and from participating in healthy relationships. Naturally this is part of our overall sense of wellness. However, this can be a challenge for some people, and especially if you are suffering persistent pain. Disrupted sleep, a change in daily activity levels, an inability to exercise, and stress will all take their toll.

People suffering from ME/CFS struggle enormously with low energy levels to put it mildly. In particular, after being active and sometimes minimally, they experience severe fatigue.

How you organise your day, planning activities (see Planning), and taking regular breaks becomes really important as does your sleep habit (see Sleep). Rest and recharge throughout the day form the basis of looking after your energy. Sometimes you put your feet up and do nothing per se, but you can also be proactive in how you seek to build your energy. Tom Rath emphasises the importance of this in his book, *Eat, Move, Sleep* (2013), which I refer to in more detail elsewhere.

In one sense, there are two different types of energy. One stems from the factors mentioned above (sleep, diet, time management) and the other from engagement with things and people that matter.

You may be able to relate to a situation when you have been feeling tired. Then a friend calls and suggests that you meet up. Suddenly you have more energy. Another common example can be seen when a marathon runner reaches the end of the race, somehow finding an extra source of juice to sprint (kind of!) to the line having struggled for the previous few miles. Where does that energy come from?

Like all other experiences, our energy level is a perception, or a guide. There is a message that we may need some fuel or rest, if not now, soon.

Recent work by Lisa Feldman-Barrett and others suggests that the brain works like an accountant, budgeting for our needs by anticipating our most likely next actions in a given environment. This is based on past experiences and is all processed in our biology in the dark. We have no conscious access to this going on, instead experiencing a perception that is the brain's best guess. For more on this predictive model, you can watch Anil Seth's TED talk.

If a person has been repeatedly exposed to a stressful environment, an expectation (biologically) builds that there is a threatening world to deal with, using energy. In other words, a frequent exposure to possible threats means that there can be a frequent budgeting for danger, even if one does not exist. Therefore, energy is being used on a just-in-case basis, but with very real effects. This is over a prolonged period of time, but similar to feeling anxious about an imagined future (based on possibilities and also perhaps past experience if something similar has happened) when you are not actually in that situation. You can be in a place where you would expect to feel great (e.g. a beach) yet your inner world is disturbed as you suffer (worry and fear).

To maintain our biology within healthy parameters, this anticipation of needs plays a key role. A simple example I use to explain this is standing up. Before you stand up, your blood pressure goes up to ensure enough oxygen is going to your brain as you change position. If there is a delay or the mechanism is ineffective, your blood pressure does not rise sufficiently and you will feel dizzy, see stars, or feel lightheaded. In severe cases, people can fall over or faint. The key is the anticipation.

As an accountant, if the budget is running low, you need to conserve energy. What uses the most energy? Moving and learning. This is why when you are tired, the thought of moving, being active, exercising, or doing something novel can feel like a chore or impossible. Your systems are on a saving mode. It means that if you do feel like doing or trying something, it's a good sign.

Sometimes people tell me that they wanted to do something different or new, they did it and then it was painful. The assumption was that they did something wrong or caused themselves an injury. This is unlikely. The pain is often a prediction based on past experience rather than what they have been doing, so no injury or harm. Additionally, when you are active, it can be sore and painful afterwards as your body adapts. I also point out that it is a good sign that they are now willing to try things and explore the world again.

Active energy management

There are two elements to active energy management: (1) planning and periodising your day into chunks with pauses in between for rest, recovery, and recharge, as already mentioned, and (2) choosing practices that lift your energy.

For the first element, see the Planning section.

On your practices to build and lift energy, what are you already doing? How successful are you? What is working for you?

To add some choices, here are some ideas from people I have worked with.

Before though, here is a question that I ask groups when we start the session: write down (or think about) five things that give you energy in your personal life, and five things in your professional life. As you are thinking of these energisers, notice how you feel in your body. Just as when we think of things that are worrying, we feel it in our body, the same happens when we think of things we love. Of course, to do this we must be present. By the way, you can of course modify the questions if you are not working; that is, five things in my life that give me energy.

As you practice focusing on these things, you get better. Can we shift our default thinking towards what is good as a lens to look at life? Yes. How far will vary from person to person and depending upon their circumstances.

Things that lift energy can include the following:

- Thinking about someone who inspires and encourages you
- Music
- Comedy
- A shower
- Being in nature
- Breathing
- Moving
- Fresh air
- A hug
- A drink
- A snack
- Thinking of a loved one
- Writing
- Doing something for someone else
- Meditation
- Mindful practice
- Feet up on the couch
- A nap (40 minutes; before mid-afternoon—only if you sleep well. If your sleep is disturbed this may interfere with your sleep drive)
- Holding hands
- Calling a friend
- Playing with the kids
- Knitting (and being creative)

Now you have made your list and added to them, these are your choices during your rest and recharge breaks.

Some of the ways you can lift your energy will also require energy. This is why making conscious choices is important, weighing up the pluses and minuses. If you have just been active and need to recoup, it will be the less active practices that help. For example, you may have been for a walk and need some recovery time. In this instance you choose a drink, to sit down, and use breathing practice. In another situation when you feel that you need a lift, you call a friend or write a poem.

You will have noticed that there are many ways to influence your energy. The ones that make the real difference are those associated with what matters to you in life—your values. If family and friends are important, then any type of connection (talking, on the phone, video call, holding hands) will feel good or better. Making value-based decisions is in line with building health and wellness.

Carving out your own way in your world can give you a sense of empowerment as you are making the choices. This is where activities that bring you pleasure and joy play a role in overcoming pain. In these states, you feel better and are able to deal with the ups and downs with more skill and clarity. Stringing these experiences together can start to change the way you feel about your situation. Being proactive also means that you start to build a feeling of self-reliance, confidence, and trust in yourself. All these are the ingredients for shaping a positive future.

Encouragement points

- Managing your energy is a proactive process that is part of your day-to-day plan.
- Rest and recharge points throughout the day need to be consistent.
- Recovery after activity allows your body to adapt to what you have been doing.
- There are many ways to manage and build your energy. You must make it individual, in line with what matters to you.

Compassion

'One compassionate word, action or thought can reduce another person's suffering and bring joy.' Thich Nhat Hahn

Compassion has been defined as 'a sensitivity to suffering in self and others with a commitment to try to alleviate and prevent it' (Gilbert, 2014).

To be compassionate is innate. It is natural to care for others and ourselves. There are plenty of examples to be seen each day. It can sound straightforward, but because of social conditioning we can find ourselves resisting.

Some will consider this to be an important area of practice in overcoming your pain. Developing a compassionate way means that you attend kindly to your needs, turning towards your suffering with courage, wisdom, and strength. Now that you have a deeper knowledge of your pain, I hope that you can understand why. In short, because compassion activates a soothing state, counter to the threat. It is a very different biology and experience that fosters health and well-being.

These are considered to be the three directional flows of compassion (Gilbert, 2010): self to others, others to self, and self to self. Often the self to others flows well. However, receiving someone else's caring concern can be more challenging. Then by far the most difficult for many people is taking the time to care for themselves, despite this being the most important. To care for others you must be well. So why might this be?

The simple answer is that you were conditioned to believe certain things about yourself from a young age. The environment in which you grew up, the type of care you received, your education, and social circumstances all played a role in shaping your beliefs, worldviews and the development of a self-critic.

Further, the way that our brains have evolved means that the human mind works in this way. One of the important first steps when coming through the compassionate lens is to accept that the way your brain and mind works is not your fault. You did not choose either, or your body or the life that you were born into. However, having given yourself a break, you soon realise that it is your responsibility to discover ways to live your best life.

The self-critic shows up in many ways from the subtle to the obvious. We all have one and we often listen. The people I work with tell me what their critic is saying when I ask them how they are doing. Examples can include: I overdid it, I was stupid, I feel so hopeless as a parent, I don't deserve to get better, I feel useless. There is very little encouragement or caring concern.

You will make mistakes. This is an essential part of learning. Unfortunately, many people feel that mistakes are somehow bad. They have learned this previously by being treated a particular way and have brought it forward. For this reason, they can live in fear of mistakes, avoiding certain situations, creating great anxiety, and sometimes trying to cover up when things go wrong. You can see how a different belief, one that fosters errors as important for growth, would bring different results. In addition, coming through a compassionate lens, there is no blame, no regret, but only forgiveness, learning, and moving on. Which feels better?

Sometimes the critic is useful as a way to think about what you have done if indeed there is some guidance. Considering how you could have done something better and setting out that intent for next time is akin to giving yourself some feedback and acting upon it.

The problem is that the self-critic, when unkind, can trigger the threat system. This has significant implications for pain, which is part of the way we protect ourselves. In thinking about yourself in an uncaring way, you move away from the practices and the ways you can feel better. You drift off the path and shift into a survival state. The brain anticipates that the world could be dangerous and mobilises systems just in case. In this state, you can experience tension, feelings of anxiety, and pain.

Another strong feeling that you learn early in life is shame. This is a powerful set of emotions in response to a perceived social threat. The instinctive fear is of rejection from the group. You have a need to be seen, valued, and loved. You want others to like you. The feeling of shame emerges when you feel others disapprove. Shaming remains a way that people treat each other. There are many examples of this in the teaching, coaching, and parenting world. Fortunately, there are better ways that are grounded in compassion.

Compassion and self-care can be considered skills to practice. Certainly, compassion can become one of the predominant ways that we live. A style or approach to life if you like. It starts with creating a compassionate self. Many argue that this version of ourselves already exists and merely needs watering.

This may seem like an alternative practice yet consider that it is completely normal to have different versions of ourselves depending on where we are and what we are doing. Our behaviour and way of being adapts accordingly. For a moment, you may like to think about how you are when at home, with friends, and at work.

There are many compassion-based practices. I have suggested a few below. It is also worth remembering that simply taking a few moments for yourself to recharge, to move, to breathe, or something else, is an act of self-compassion.

If some of these things trigger a strong response, you may benefit from speaking to a trained therapist so that you can obtain the help you need.

Self-caring

Looking after yourself takes many forms, including the practices of self-compassion. The first step is to take the time for yourself, even in short bursts, so that you can care for others in the way that you want.

Practices

1. A simple question to yourself: recognising that this situation is difficult and painful, what is something I can do right now that would be most helpful?
2. A self-compassion brief break: (1) recognise that this is a moment of suffering—using your own words, name the problem or acknowledge that it is really hard (2) acknowledge that suffering is a part of life; it is normal, part of being human and many people are facing hard situations (3) may I be kind to myself at this moment. To think about how you would care for and speak to a friend or loved one gives you a guide.
3. Creating and building the compassionate self: by practising the compassionate self, as suggested by the Compassionate Mind Foundation, you have a state that you can slip into when needed. You can start by listening to their recording on Soundcloud.
4. The practice of self-compassion or metta meditation (loving-kindness): this is something you can practise regularly to water your own seeds of compassion, for yourself, and others. There are many resources you can use. For example, on Kristen Neff's (an assistant professor at The University of Texas) website are a range of practices, the Waking Up and Ten Percent apps. You will also find many YouTube videos. The key is to find a practice that works for you—some voices resonate more than others. The essence of this practice is to use certain phrases when you direct your loving-kindness to others and yourself. Whilst this can feel uncomfortable initially, the effects are powerful. And you don't even need to feel any great emotion for there to be a change in your behaviour. Research now suggests that the loving-kindness practice is a skill that can be cultivated to make us happier and more resourceful. Think of the importance of that for overcoming pain. Compassion and loving-kindness are strengths.

Making metta part of your routine means that you are consistently self-caring and nourishing the compassionate part of you, bolstering to work with other parts of you that are more tricky. As the self-critic is often so strong in the people I work with, this creates a practical way forward.

Encouragement points

- Compassion is the antidote to suffering.
- The compassionate part of you is self-soothing, which is an important skill and way to respond to moments of suffering.

- We can practise specific skills to nurture the compassionate self.
- Building a metta practice into your routine is a way of consistently practising taking care of yourself.
- Many people want to care for others, but this starts with caring for and being compassionate towards yourself.

Talking to yourself

'To stop and communicate with yourself is a revolutionary act.' Thich Nhat Hanh

We each have an inner voice that we are more or less aware of at different times. This voice has a range of tones and agendas, using a particular style of language and chosen words. The impact of this voice can be enormous, influencing our mood, the decisions we make, and how we perceive ourselves and the world. Perhaps there is nothing more powerful, and hence the importance of understanding your voice and harnessing its potential.

It requires a presence of mind to be aware of what you are thinking rather than being caught up in the thought. Some talk of creating some space between the thinker (you) and the thought. Understanding and knowing that you are not your thoughts is an important realisation. Becoming entangled with thoughts and the inseparable emotions (they come together as you will notice when you examine your own experience) takes you away from the present moment, whereas to know that you are thinking puts you in the privileged position of seeing things for what they are. You realise the impermanent nature of things and how they are always changing, even if the sense of you feels the same. What we are telling ourselves about what is happening, and what is actually happening are often different.

A good example of this in relation to pain is when you tell yourself or others, 'it is the same'.

This is your thought and it is a real one—thoughts are always real. You believe this to be the nature of your experience and the truth of the matter. But, the actual truth, and perhaps a painful one, is that things are never the same. There is constant change afoot. No moment or experience of that moment has ever been before and will ever be again. Life would not be possible if this were not the case. This gives great hope.

You might like to try this if you become aware of this kind of dialogue. Look at the circumstances. Are they really the same? For this to be true, time would have to stand still. You could say that the story you are telling is the same. But even that is not exactly the same because it is a different moment.

One problem is that your memory is not an exact representation of what happened before. It is just good enough, and each time you recall, there is a slight change or update according to the current circumstances. In essence, it is just a guide. For sure, you cannot remember exactly what it felt like yesterday or even a few minutes ago. You may know that you felt pain, but you cannot recall that pain as it was. The version you experience now is just that, now, and not then.

This may sound like I am playing with words, but there is an importance because of the stories you tell yourself and their influence on your lived experience. They are literally playing a role in shaping your experiences. This is why there is a skill to be learned and practised when it comes to the inner voice.

Distinct yet related are the ways you talk to yourself and others. Fortunately, you can cultivate and practise a way of communicating in both forms, which is compassionate. Thich Nhat Hanh (2013) describes four guidelines of the Ten Bodhisattva Trainings for Right Speech:

1. Tell the truth
2. Don't exaggerate
3. Be consistent
4. Use peaceful language

To tell the truth, you must know the truth. This is why understanding your pain and symptoms is pivotal, both the science (the depth can vary from person to person) and the experience. To get close to the truth of the matter, you take your knowledge and apply it to what is happening right now, giving meaning and validation to the feeling. From there you can decide your next best action. A further ingredient is presence.

A truth about pain that you have known for many years is that the experience relates poorly to the extent of the injury, tissue damage, or inflammatory process (see section Pain truths). Pat Wall, one of the fathers of pain medicine, wrote and spoke of this in 1979. Despite this being known for 50 years, the predominant model remains focused on searching for a structural or anatomical reason for pain. There isn't one! And now you know about pain (see section What is pain?), you know the truth.

When others ask you about your pain, you can tell the truth. The level of explanation can vary of course. Some people have different scripts for different situations. Knowing that you have these to hand (not literally!), means you can feel more confident, rather than worrying about what you will say. The answer you give to a close friend is different to a work colleague or stranger. You will decide what is appropriate. Of course, there are times when you may wish to protect someone from the reality of your suffering, for instance, a child. This is not an easy decision. You may choose to say that you are fine, but it is likely your body signals, facial expression, and how you were before they asked (observable—which is maybe why they asked) are giving away something else. There is nothing wrong with pausing to create a little space before answering.

One way of answering questions about your pain that some people find helpful is to start by acknowledging the question: that is, thanks for asking. You can then lead the way. In other words, the way you reply leads the conversation and how they then respond. A possibility opens up, allowing you to say that you are in pain, but that you are working on various things to move forward. This gives it a positive edge to focus on and to allow the other person to encourage you as well as to empathise. In many cases, people want empathy rather than solutions—as humans we do like to be helpful and offer suggestions; my friend went to see … have you tried …? and so on. Whatever response you give and the way you deliver it will elicit a further response from the other person. What kind of responses do you want? Answering this question will give you insights into what you might say.

Closely tied to speaking the truth is to refrain from exaggerating. Of course, if we are telling the truth, there is no exaggeration! There are plenty of ways that sensory data can be amplified within our biological systems. We don't need to add to this unnecessarily.

There may be a temptation to do this for several reasons. The most common of these is to be heard. By embellishing the story or the description of the feelings, there is a need to be acknowledged when this has perhaps not been forthcoming. Many people suffering persistent pain have told me that they have not been taken seriously, they have been dismissed or even disbelieved. Of course, this tells us that the person listening to the descriptions (if indeed they are listening as opposed to imposing their own thoughts) does not understand pain. This is a huge problem as there can be little progress without a meaning being given to the pain and the story being validated.

Some people need empathy and want to feel supported by people close by. It is understandable then to talk of pain and suffering greater than is actually experienced. Of course, it is hard to measure, so people will respond in different ways. The person feeling pain may want some kind of specific help or for someone else to do something for them, and so it becomes more likely they will offer it if the pain is described as worse in some cases. Repeated conversations about pain can also send people the other way. Undoubtedly, persistent pain adds significant pressure to relationships (see section Family and friends).

The major problem with exaggerating the symptoms is not actually in how it impacts others. It is more about how it impacts the speaker. We create our perceptions using thoughts, emotions, expectations, feelings, attention, and more. Hence, by amplifying the current state of pain, you are actually impacting upon your very experience of pain. The experience is not limited to the intensity, the description, and the embodied location, but it includes the context, how you see the world, what you are able to do, and your connections with people and society to name but a few. There is a much bigger picture at play.

So, the things you say to others are also impacting on you. This is why having a selection of scripts that can guide different conversations can be helpful.

This can also work the other way. For instance, in a therapy session a person may say that they are better to please the therapist, when in fact this is not the case. The reasons for this go beyond this guide, but are important to address if they come up. You can see how this would also relate closely to telling the truth or not, for some kind of gain.

I want to add a caveat before continuing. With this and some of the other topics, I am aware that it can sound like the person, you, are being blamed for these behaviours and actions. Having read my comments on compassion and coming through this lens, the starting point is exactly the opposite. It is not the fault of the person for the way they think. This has resulted from prior social conditioning and circumstances. They have not chosen their mind. But when there is a realisation about what is actually happening, there is a responsibility to learn and do things in a better way.

Consistently speaking the truth in a compassionate manner reinforces to you and to others what is happening for you and where you are going. You lead the way. Consistency also means that what you say to different people is similar, not trying to gain any advantage from one person over another. It is about being true to your word, and not just in relation to your pain and suffering, but in all that you say. Communication is an art, and a powerful one.

Just as you need to be consistent with our practices of exercise, self-compassion, and caring to be healthy, you can also be this way with your speech. There is the ripple effect to consider, which is the knock-on effect of the way you are with someone and how they then treat the next person—this can go both ways of course. You build people's confidence in you as someone who delivers as they promise; you are reliable. This develops trust and stronger connections which are an important part of being well.

Using peaceful language acts as a way of creating safety to connect, acts as a balm in stressful situations, and is self-soothing. You 'hear' everything that you say. In a sense, this ties the four guidelines together. Peaceful and calming words spoken consistently, truthfully, and accurately bring us together, validate each other, and offer hope. When someone is suffering, to receive and ingest the words, 'I hear you', can be hugely impacting.

If I employ peaceful language, it changes my perception. Wittgenstein said: 'The limits of my language means the limits of my world.' He implies that for something to exist for us, you must have the language to describe it. To speak and to think in language are actions that shape the world you experience. In terms of pain then, your perceptions in part are generated through the words you use. Again, you are using the words to yourself (you hear them), reinforcing some evidence you have of pain and suffering, and to others who in turn reflect back empathy or something else. You are immersed in the interaction, which is the context for the pain. This context is also part of the pain experience—where you are embedded. You will now see how you can positively influence your own experiences by noticing and perhaps changing your language to reflect where you are going rather than where you have been.

For example, changing the descriptions you use. Instead of burning pain, you say a warm feeling. You might argue that this is not what you are feeling, it is burning. Indeed, this may be true of the moment. But where do you want to go? Much as you would point your car where you want to go, you do the same with your intent via words. Further, the word pain can be replaced with soreness or discomfort. Then you gently observe any embodied effects.

Communication is at the heart of many important parts of life. My encouragement to you is to develop self-coaching skills so that you can make the best choices as often as possible, thereby achieving results. This is one of those skills that you can practise and improve. Listening to yourself, acknowledging the different parts of you that conflict (self-critic, self-carer), being present, and then choosing peaceful, truthful words consistently will keep you on the right path.

Asking yourself appreciative questions

These are questions you can skilfully ask yourself to direct your thinking and actions. At the heart is an appreciation of your strengths and potential as an individual. The purpose is to get the best of yourself.

Here are some examples. If you decide to practise, I encourage you to notice how you feel when you ask yourself the question.

- What has gone well today?
- Previously when faced with a challenge, what strengths did I use to be successful?
- What is my best decision right now?
- What can I do here and now?
- How can I approach today in the best way?

What did you notice?

Where did the question put your attention?

You can of course come up with your own questions depending on your circumstances and what you want to achieve. These are questions you can also ask of others to appreciate them as human beings who are also trying to do their best with the skills and knowledge that they have.

Encouragement points

- The person we talk to the most is ourselves.
- How do you talk to yourself? Kindly? Patiently? With compassion? Or something else?
- How could you talk to yourself that would be encouraging?
- What kinds of questions can you ask yourself that appreciate your strengths?
- How would you talk to someone you care about? Then do the same to yourself.
- You can train yourself to talk kindly to yourself—it is a skill to practise.

Mindfulness and meditation

'Mindfulness and meditation practices are practical ways to see things as they really are rather than the distortions of the mind.' RS

Mindfulness meditation and other meditative practices have become popular in Western society. Often, they are described as a way to relax, be calm, and present, which can sound appealing. However, it is more accurate to think of mindfulness as a way of being. It is not just about sitting and breathing, and the purpose is certainly not to get anywhere. In fact, it is quite the opposite.

You are trying to be in the here and now, open to whatever is happening. Rather than resisting, fighting, avoiding, or ignoring. To transform your experience, you must be open, acceptant, and practise letting go. This is not what we are trained to do so it can feel counterintuitive.

To be present means you can be aware of what is happening, what you are thinking and doing. If you are not present, instead lost in thoughts about the future or the past, you cannot see what is happening. Spending time in the now, which is the only time, is really living. You are awake and experiencing the full richness of life, whatever this is like for you. This moment is the one for healing because it is the only one. Taking care of now is taking care of your future. This is both a philosophical position and a practical one that becomes available through mindful practice.

You have preferences. Some things you like and some things you don't. You try to hold onto the things you like and punch away those you don't. You continually try to shape and control the world according to your preferences. If this is you, you are trying to control the uncontrollable. Life is happening regardless of your preferences and there is nothing you or anyone can do about that.

Sounds harsh? I don't mean it this way. It is the reality of course. Having this insight means you can be more accepting of what is happening and focus on what you can control: your approach and responses to life's circumstances. In turn, you can go about creating the conditions for your better, healthier, happier future.

'Happiness is not something ready made. It comes from your own actions', Dalia Lama XIV

One of the pioneering teachers of mindfulness and peace for living well in our world was Thich Nhat Hanh, a Vietnamese Zen Master who recently passed away (January 2022). Or as he put it, his continuation. In other words, he continues through his community, in their actions. These can also be your actions. The teachings have been passed down to his students, both monastics and lay-people to continue his work in engaged Buddhism.

'I am a continuation, like the rain is a continuation of a cloud', Thich Nhat Hanh

Thay, as he was affectionately known by his students, spoke of mindfulness as an energy for compassion to be practised through the day, not only in sitting meditation. It is a path or a way of living that is in the here and now. Each step you take along that path can bring happiness and joy. On happiness, which we have been encouraged to seek and find in our society, Thay said concisely:

'There is no way to happiness—happiness is the way.' He also famously asked the question, 'Does it make you happy?'. This is something we can ponder ourselves silently.

Mindfulness practice is grounded in the Dhamma, or teachings of the Buddha. I will point out here that I am not seeking to convert you to Buddhism. That is not the purpose of this section. I am not a Buddhist but have found the principles to be helpful both professionally and personally.

Instead, it is for you to understand that there are practical ways of applying the principles so that you can shape a positive future: helpful insights. This was the work of Thich Nhat Hanh who was a proponent of engaged Buddhism, a particular form dedicated to positive social change. You can think of the principles as guidance rather than a doctrine, much like this book. A guide on the side.

Together with the practice of mindfulness, having an understanding of Buddhist principles can be useful, but is not absolutely necessary to gain the benefits. To deepen your understanding, I would suggest reading The Miracle of Mindfulness and Peace is Every Step by Thich Nhat Hanh. You can also visit the Plum Village website where you will find written and recorded teachings, many practices, and a podcast.

Below I have shared a brief explanation of the Four Noble Truths and the Noble Eightfold Path so you can gain a flavour of the underpinnings.

The four noble truths

1. Life always involves suffering.
2. The cause of this suffering is craving (desire) and ignorance (misunderstanding of the truth of reality that we are separate, and so we maintain the illusion of self).
3. There is an end to suffering when we awaken.
4. By living a particular way, including practicing mindfulness, and gaining and using wisdom, we can wake up and become enlightened.

The noble eightfold path

1. Right understanding
2. Right thought
3. Right speech
4. Right action
5. Right livelihood

6. Right effort
7. Right mindfulness
8. Right concentration

These eight factors work together to promote ethical and moral conduct, mental discipline, and wisdom. This is considered to be the path to freedom or the end of suffering. Much has been written about each.

Taking right speech as an example, this refers to avoiding any kind of harmful speech. Talking behind people's backs, gossiping, bringing disharmony and division by what you say, using hateful, rude, or abusive language are all examples. When you put this out into the world, it is reflected back, causing disturbance and suffering for others and yourself. This may not be immediate.

To gain a better sense of mindfulness as a way of being, here are some quotes from Thich Nhat Hanh.

My encouragement to you: take your time to read each and consider the meaning.

'With mindfulness, you can establish yourself in the present in order to touch the wonders of life that are available in that moment.'

'Many people are alive but don't touch the miracle of being alive.'

'Drink your tea slowly and reverently, as if it is the axis on which the whole earth revolves—slowly, evenly, without rushing toward the future. Live the actual moment. Only this moment is life.'

'We have the tendency to run away from suffering and to look for happiness. But, in fact, if you have not suffered, you have no chance to experience real happiness.'

'Buddhism teaches us not to try to run away from suffering. You have to confront suffering. You have to look deeply into the nature of suffering in order to recognise its cause, the making of the suffering.'

'Most of us experience a life full of wonderful moments and difficult moments. But for many of us, even when we are most joyful, there is fear behind our joy.'

'Fearlessness is not only possible, it is the ultimate joy. When you touch non-fear, you are free.'

Awareness

'It is in our awareness and our capacity to pay attention that the potential for healing and transformation in relationship to our pain resides.' Jon Kabat-Zinn (2023).

Put simply, being aware of something is a different experience from being caught up in it. Awareness of being in pain is different from being in pain. Your awareness cannot be in pain—ask yourself, is my awareness in pain?

This is a simple shift. Changing how you relate to your pain changes your pain. I say simple, that's the principle. It takes practice, and meditation is the practice.

The practice of mindfulness

In the ideal world, you would learn to practice with a teacher. Next best is via a high-quality app such as the Plum Village app, Ten Percent, or Waking Up by Sam Harris. These apps offer excellent instructions and teachings. To practice mindfulness, you also need some understanding of Buddhist psychology as outlined above. It is easy to stray from the path otherwise.

I will share a couple of basic practices (below). In essence they appear to be simple. However, when you try you will see what it is actually like to try to be present with a mind that seems to like to wander.

I suggest and encourage mindfulness practice (or at least try it for a while) to the people I work with so that they can examine their own experiences. To see what is really going on and get a better grip on the world. The practice that enables being more present and aware means that you can respond more and more skilfully to whatever life presents to you.

The clarity and inner calmness you cultivate allow you to make better and better decisions. You also see and live in a different world when inner peace becomes your way. What is happening inside of you biologically and how it feels is influencing how you see the world and how you see yourself in that world. It all comes as one experience, which you will start to see with your practice.

Mindfulness naturally allows you to see things as they are more closely, which can differ from your thoughts. Realising the difference between what you are actually experiencing (the raw feelings) and your interpretation (the story about the feelings) is very important. What you are feeling, you are feeling. That is your reality. There is nothing you can do about it because it is already there and happening to you. The way you interpret what you are feeling and how you then respond is what you can control. One of the most important insights.

Psychiatrist, psychotherapist, and author Mark Epstein MD offers many important insights. Here are a couple to consider:

'When we stop distancing ourselves from the pain in the world, our own or others', we create the possibility of a new experience, one that often surprises because of how much joy, connection, or relief it yields.'

'Awakening does not mean a change in difficulty, it means a change in how those difficulties are met.'

There are thousands and thousands of insights from different traditions and thinkers. Of course, you will find your own that resonate, which I encourage you to seek out. They can become your daily mantras and guiding lights, especially when the path becomes windy and dimly lit.

Many people are doing better than they think, but this can be obscured by a strong narrative that says something else. The stories we tell ourselves are very powerful and convincing but are often not true. Similarly with memories, which we know are updated each time we retrieve them. They are a best guess about what happened, with many gaps and dependent on how we are feeling in the moment we are thinking about them. There is plenty of room for distortion. Meditation practice allows you to examine this closely and get a better grip as well as disrupt sticky beliefs that are limiting your progress.

Gaining clarity and presence, we are able to make best and better decisions.

A question that pops up is why would you want to sit or be with your own suffering? Or, why would I want to face the difficult and unpleasant feelings? This is a good question, especially, in a society that encourages us to be distracted or turn away from things that are painful, to indulge in only pleasure, and to pursue our desires. The problem with this approach is that you don't have the opportunity to soothe your suffering by avoiding it.

Naturally to be present when you are suffering takes courage, understanding, and self-compassion, all of which you have.

You may have come across the idea of becoming comfortable with being uncomfortable. As you know, life is full of challenges, ups and downs, aches, and pains. Certainties are ageing, disease, and death. Sounds grim! But it is true. Turning it around, knowing these are definite, we can appreciate what is happening and what we have right now. Accepting truisms is an important part of easing your own suffering. So instead of trying to control life and avoid the bumps in the road, you can accept them as the norm and learn skills to deal with them.

Some people find that this is an effective way to grow and lead a richer life. This may not hold an appeal at first sight, but with difficulties being part of our existence, you can either learn to deal with them better and better or suffer more by resisting. There is the choice.

How will you relate to each moment? How will you relate to what is happening?

So, to the process of waking up and learning to be present to ease your own suffering.

Below are some common practices to help you start. If you have your own preferred teachers or resources, you may still like to read through them.

Remember that these are skills to learn. Each time you sit or lie and practise is a step. It is not the end result—process over prize. It is like learning a language or musical instrument. A route of mastery rather than there being an outcome, along which you gain insights that help you see things as they are, navigate life skilfully, and ease your own suffering.

Being a practice, consistency matters as with all the skills and strategies in the book. Interwoven into your life and day.

Breathing awareness

Sitting upright and relaxed if you can, try to maintain a small arch in your lower back. Notice what it is like to be sitting, feeling how the chair or the floor is supporting your body.

Next, bring your attention to your breathing. Where do you feel it the most? It could be your nose, your chest, or tummy. Gently keep your attention here as you breathe in and out, without trying to control or change the way you are breathing. You are simply paying attention to your breath.

Some people find it helpful to use a mantra or phrase to stay present. For instance, breathing in, I am aware I am breathing in. Breathing out, I am aware I am breathing out. After a few cycles, breathing in, breathing out. Or just in, out. This is a practice encouraged by Thich Nhat Hanh.

As you practise, you may notice how you drop into a deeper sense of calm without trying to adjust your breathing pattern.

This practice can be brief and repeated throughout the day. Setting a notification like the Mindful Bell from the Plum Village app will remind you to pause and become aware of 2-3 breaths. You could set this hourly. At other times, you may practise for longer.

Breathing awareness is also a way to skilfully respond to painful and challenging moments. You could think of it as applying the brakes.

It is inevitable that whilst you are practising, your mind will wander. You will be distracted by sounds, thoughts, feelings, and other interruptions. When this happens, you can acknowledge whatever it was, and then gently bring your attention back to your breathing. You can think of this as training to refocus, which is an important part of living mindfully.

Many people give up or feel that they are failing because they cannot clear their mind or stop thinking. They believe that they must be doing it wrong if their mind goes off. This is not true. This is part of the practice. If you persevere, you will find that you notice this more and more, and address it skilfully.

Body scan

You can practise the body scan sitting or lying. If you decide to lie down though, there is a chance you may fall asleep. That is fine, you probably need the rest. But it is not practice.

A body scan is a simple way of connecting with your body, an important part of being healthy and whole. This can be a challenge when the body is the perceived source of suffering or doubt. Yet we need to make that connection, accepting all parts of ourselves as one.

The practice is simple in concept. You may like to read the instructions first and then have a go.

Once you have chosen your position, close your eyes and become aware of what it is like to be lying or sitting. You may like to take a few easy breaths to be present and focused.

Now take your attention to your head and notice all the feelings, including nothing at all! Then pass your attention down your face, down your neck, across your shoulders, down one arm to your hand and each finger. Now down your other arm to your hand and each finger. Just noticing whatever appears, and passes by.

Continue down your chest and tummy, down your back to your hips and pelvis. There may be places you like to pause and breathe. Down one leg to your knee, to your ankle, foot, and toes. Then down the other leg, to your knee, ankle, foot, and toes.

Having scanned down your whole body, now expand your awareness to take in your whole body and notice whatever appears in your consciousness.

Finally, you can practise breathing awareness, coming back to the room, checking in to how you are feeling and noting any changes in state.

The body scan can be practised in a matter of seconds or minutes or longer.

Open awareness

Instead of focusing on your breath, in this practice you are open to whatever appears in your awareness. You let it in and you let it pass by, as it will if you don't interfere with it.

So, what is 'it'? It could be a thought, a feeling, a sound, a sensation, or anything else that you become aware of. You will start to notice how all these things appear without you doing anything in particular. Take sounds for instance. Become aware of any sounds where you are right now. There's nothing you need to do to hear them.

The practice of open awareness helps you develop the skill of being present and allowing whatever is happening to happen without interference. It is happening anyway. When you realise that you don't have to react and you can choose what to respond to and how it becomes very empowering. You are focusing on what you can control rather than what you can't. This feels good—success.

You could think of this as a way to roll with life as it unfolds, developing equanimity. This is a balanced and calm mind, which you can practise in order to meet all people and circumstances. It does not mean that you do not feel the full set of emotional states. Indeed, you do but with full awareness, and without the reactivity and additional suffering caused by the way you think about it.

As things arise in your awareness and you notice, there will be judgement and reference to preferences. I am not sure if we can ever be without judgement as it forms part of how we relate to life. Of course, judgement can be wrong, and often is! This can cause problems. Becoming aware of your judgements means that you can skilfully decide whether this thought is useful or accurate rather than be entangled and act as if this is the only possibility and truth. Of course, it isn't in most cases.

A couple of useful questions:

1. This thought I am having, it is real but is it true?
2. Is this thought useful?

A practice within open awareness and as you live moment to moment is labelling. This creates some space for better responses. One of the key insights is that it is not the situation, it's the way you respond that matters. Labelling allows you to pull back, experience a change in state, and then make your next best decision.

If you feel pain, for example, you can say to yourself: 'there is pain'. Similarly with tension, anxiety, or any other feeling. This little bit of distance offers an opportunity to notice what is happening for you, clarify your needs, and then choose an action that best meets your needs.

Rumination is a common experience for many people. Recurring thoughts, pondering on the same subject over and over. It can be overwhelming. And, of course, with the mind being embodied, you feel it. This affects how you move, how the world appears to you in terms of possibilities, and your emotional state. These are entwined of course. Labelling in this case can be a helpful skill. Saying gently to yourself: 'thinking, thinking, thinking', again pulls you back, enabling you to see things for what they are.

To practise open awareness, you sit upright and relaxed. You can have your eyes open or closed. Notice your body and the different sensations as they appear and disappear. It is like you are watching a film in the cinema. Or some describe it like watching clouds float across the sky. Whatever works for you. Then become aware of your breathing, following it in, and out for a few moments. Next you can just be aware of whatever arises, no controlling, just letting it go.

You may find it helpful to set a time to begin. Just a few minutes—set the bar low so that you set yourself up for a win. Remember that if your mind wanders, you haven't done anything wrong. That's what your mind is really good at! When you notice that you have become caught up in thinking, acknowledge the thought (or label), and then drop back into being openly aware. Repeat.

Loving-kindness

Loving-kindness is the simple practice of repeating certain phrases to yourself as a way of offering a gift to yourself and others. What is that gift? The clue is in the title, but what does this mean?

You offer well-wishing and caring concern accompanied by an action (the act of saying the phrases with meaning), so full of compassion. In doing this, you are cultivating a different and kindly way to meet life, other people, and yourself. Many people find caring for others to be very natural and easy, but when kindness is turned towards them, it becomes uncomfortable.

Being kind towards oneself does not come naturally to many people, but is essential for getting and feeling better.

In chronic pain, the critical self poses a problem in different ways. Notably, it can mean not enough self-care as well as being hard on yourself for not reaching a bar that has been set too high.

'I should be able to …' is a common cry. The question is whether this is in line with reality or not. Or, 'I should be better by now. What is wrong with me?'

There are plenty of variations and often quite subtle. You may not even notice if you are being unnecessarily hard on yourself or unfair. Fortunately, the loving-kindness practice can help.

Sitting upright and relaxed with your eyes open or closed, feel your body in sitting. Take a few easy breaths to be present and focused. Now repeat the following phrases: may I be safe, may I be healthy, may I be happy, may I live with ease. To start, you can do this for a few minutes, perhaps using a timer. As you become more familiar, you can increase the time.

Importantly, you don't need to feel strong emotions. The fact that you are trying and that you have the right intent is enough.

The practice can then be extended to someone you know well: may you be safe, may you be healthy, may you be happy, may you live with ease. The following two steps use the same phrases directed towards someone you know vaguely and then someone who you find to be mildly annoying. Mildly. Five minutes of practice towards yourself and the others would be a good starting point.

Naturally I cannot tell you what your experience will be like. You will discover for yourself. The types of things people who practise describe include feeling generally happier, acting more generously, being more patient with themselves and others, and relating to situations more calmly. If this were you, do you think this would help you relate to your pain differently and respond more skilfully? Also taking care of your self-critic.

If you prefer to listen and be guided through the practice, there are many videos online. In particular, look out for Sharon Salzberg and Kristen Neff for loving-kindness meditations.

Being with your pain

The way to transform any experience is by facing it, being open to what is happening, and allowing it to pass. It always will because this is the true nature of things—impermanence. If you are feeling pain at this moment, the circumstances are such that this is the only experience you could be having. Knowing and accepting this helps you to see things as they truly are rather than the story you are telling yourself.

Cultivating such openness takes know-how and practice. Particularly if you are wondering why you would sit with your pain when it is the very thing you don't want! The common coping skills that people use are to avoid, limit, restrict, distract, or numb. This can bring short-term relief from the pain or from the thought of doing something painful There is a reward in avoidance! But, this does not lead to any sustained transformation or freedom from suffering.

This is similar to other fears and concerns. Take a fear of spiders. You can do everything that you can to avoid spiders, which takes effort and limits your possibilities. You may decide that it is worth it of course. But one day, you are very likely to meet a spider because the reality is you cannot control life and what it presents to you. Now what do you do?

Without having learned ways to reduce your fear and skills to deal with your emotions and the situation, you are ill-equipped. The alternative is to face the fear little by little and build your skills and hence confidence to move forward and experience freedom.

Through meditation practice you learn to notice the difference between the raw experiences you are having and the story you tell yourself. Within the space between comes the opportunity for you to respond more skilfully. Labelling can help.

When you notice your pain, you can say to yourself: 'there is pain'. Next, you can examine the feelings more closely, learning that there are nuanced sensations and experiences within that disrupt the idea that it is just pain and is always there in the same way.

You are disrupting what you thought was happening and then repairing it to make it better, which means suffering less. Getting better and overcoming pain needs understanding, patience, compassion (or kindness), and is typically a step-by-step journey. Wanting to be at the end of it and pain-free is an understandable thought, but distracts you from reality. Being in reality is another key part of getting better.

Your practice

Having decided to practice mindfulness, you can create a daily habit (see Habits section). One way of doing this is to schedule a certain time (great if it is the same time each day), and then have moments of being mindful throughout the day. The effects of practice become apparent at a point in time. This is difficult to describe as each person will have their own experience. I would say that mine is to be more present and awake, meaning that I can somehow be aware of my thinking rather than get caught up with it so often. I am able to see patterns of thought and notice what is really happening instead of being wrapped up in interpretations and rumination.

There is no end to the practice, as it is a way of being. There is no goal. In essence, we don't practice to get anywhere or to be a particular type of person. We practice to be awakened to the full richness of life in this moment, the only moment, open to whatever is happening for you.

As I said at the beginning of this section, it is best to have some instruction with mindful practice and an appreciation of the underlying philosophy. It can be unusual in Western society to consider practicing without the purpose of gaining something. There are benefits to practice of course, but if you are focusing on these, you are distracted from what you are doing. Wanting to be anywhere or anything other than how things actually are right now causes suffering. A mindful practice helps you be closer to reality, cultivate clarity, equanimity and calm.

Encouragement points

- Mindfulness is a way of being.
- A daily practice of mindfulness helps you to be more present and see things for what they really are in life, including responding more skilfully to challenging moments (less reactive, more responsive).
- Ideally you find a teacher, but alternatively you can use an app such as Waking Up, Plum Village, or Healthy Minds.
- You can practise for a few minutes a day and create a habit. The time may build, but the key is consistency.
- Pausing and being mindful throughout the day help create a sense of calm and clarity.

Friends and family

'Loved ones and friends often want to help but don't know how. When they have ways to work with you, it can make an enormous difference.' RS

The people who are close by usually want to help. But often they don't know how, which can lead to different responses: for example, frustration, irritation, being over-zealous, doing too much for you, or doing too little. When I talk to the people who come to see me about their support network, we identify what works and what does not. Then you can put into place some practical strategies to make sure that everyone is moving in the same direction, encouraging you and helping when necessary.

Whilst there can be people who are willing to support you, it is not always easy to ask for help. If you value your independence, you want to be able to do things for yourself. It is frustrating and upsetting when you can't, but even so, you may try and find it is too difficult or painful. You feel worse and often the self-critic joins in to add another layer of suffering. The tussle between what you are able to do and want to do and the way you think and feel about the situation pushes and pulls you in different directions. But there is a way out and forward.

Before that, I would like to share the insight of interbeing, a word created by Thich Nhat Hanh. Essentially, we are all in this together. There is not the separation that there may appear to be. For instance, you exist because of other people. You develop your sense of who you are through other people. People share the common desire to live a happy and healthy life. There is an interconnectedness of all things. True independence does not exist in reality.

You may think that to get yourself dressed is independence. Or to go to the shop to buy a pint of milk. Yet to do these things you need others. Who made your clothes? Who delivered the milk? Who cared for the cows that produced the milk?

Acceptance of your current limitations is the opposite to the fight or resistance (see Acceptance). This is not easy for many people, but it is possible and hugely beneficial in moving onwards. In fact, it may be essential. Acceptance is not giving in as is commonly thought. Instead, it is about acknowledging where you are right now to allow you to move on. On the other hand, to resist is to increase the anguish and tension. This does take work and practice and varies day to day. It is a way of being rather than an act at a single point in time. Accepting and letting go releases you from whatever is holding you back; the stuckness. Typically, it is a story that is held onto and replayed, which is so convincing. And felt in the body.

What difference does it make to be accepting? To accept means that you can make the best choice at that moment. For instance, in your current state, you may be unable to go shopping as you want. You do need some help. There are things you can do, but some things you can't. To resist this means you either don't go shopping at all, you ask someone to do the whole job, or try and force yourself to do it. Of course, none of these options are in line with your picture of success (getting better) or what matters to you (values).

Not going shopping means you have no food, so that is not an option. Asking someone to do it for you means you miss the opportunity to practise moving and engaging with a task. There could also be an element of avoidance. Trying to force yourself to do it is likely to cause more pain and if you are unable to complete the shop, you will feel further frustration and disappointment. Within these scenarios, there is plenty of material for the self-critic to jump on to make things feel worse.

So, what can you do? The first step of acceptance means that you are open to your position and the possibilities. You can think about the parts you can be involved with and how you can participate. Then the kind of help you need becomes clear. Asking for that help can still be difficult of course, but what kinds of opportunities arise from such a request?

We are designed to co-operate. It is how we evolved and have been successful as human beings. We like to help each other. There is such a phenomenon as the helper's high. Think about a time when someone has asked you for help and you have stepped up to lend a hand. How did it feel? It is common that people who don't like to ask are often the ones who are readily available to help others.

Bearing this in mind, when you ask someone to help you, there is now an opportunity for them to feel good about what they are doing. You are giving them the chance to boost their health and sense of worth. From co-operation also comes a time to deepen bonds as you create a story together, growing and strengthening the relationship.

By accepting what you can do now and then doing this in the best way, you can build on. You now know that this is an important part of getting better. Using the word 'yet' can be a useful addition, when you think of what it is you want to do: I can't … (activity), yet. This shows that you accept where you are, but you have the intent to keep improving. Most powerful of all, you are giving this message to yourself.

Once you have shifted your position on asking for help, you establish what that help looks like. Essentially, it fills the gaps as you seek to progress your level of participation and skill. As with many of the practices that involve other people, you will usually find that you lead the way. Friends and family want to know what they can do and how. Giving this some thought can be useful before you have the conversation.

There does seem to be a tendency to see pain as a problem to fix. Or that you somehow need fixing as a person. Neither is true. With the help you receive, you are creating the conditions for a better life. That is a very different approach and in line with what we know about pain and health. If people think that you have a problem, many will jump in with a solution. They may suggest that you do something a particular way, or that they do something, and of course the recommendations are based on their own experiences or others they know. You should go and see …, or, have you tried …?, or, my friend … (did something) and it really helped; and other variations of well-meaning offerings. That is all well and good, but you may not have asked for ideas. Instead, what you wanted and needed was to be heard and validated. Perhaps a hug or a kind word would have been done.

Suggestion or empathy? Some people find it useful to clarify what they need at the moment so that the family member or friend can meet that need. This avoids frustration, irritation, and other emotions that emerge from a mismatch. Once you are feeling better, there may be a place for a suggestion. Professor Stephen Rollnick, co-founder of motivational interviewing, once said in a workshop I was attending, you knock on the door and wait to be asked in. You don't then enter and start rearranging the furniture.

In other words, we ask a question, how are you? The person answers and we listen to what they say. We can then respond with empathy, affirming their experience of suffering. We don't plough in by telling them what to do! This is the spirit of motivational interviewing that informs a skilful and compassionate way of communicating.

I have encouraged you to make a plan that you can follow each day. You can share your plan with family and friends, explaining what you are trying to achieve and how. From there you can highlight the areas that you need help with. There may be certain people who are better positioned to assist with particular jobs due to their availability, willingness, and skill level. Once everyone knows their role, it can often be easier to move forward. This also addresses the tendency for some people to do too much for you, meaning that you miss opportunities to become more skilful and independent.

Over the years, people have brought friends and family into their sessions for different reasons. For example, to be an extra pair of eyes and ears, to help explain the story, for support, and to learn how they can be helpful. This is an opportunity to explain your pain and symptoms, to deepen their understanding of your pain and the ways you are trying to move forward. The aim is to increase the engagement in the useful practices and ways that they can support you.

One of the common questions is about touch. When there is great sensitivity to touch (allodynia), people close by can be hesitant or nervous about touching you. Stroking, massage, and hugs, which can all have a role, become a problem. Understanding what is happening and how to best use these different forms of touch can be useful for soothing and showing caring, but also as a means of maintaining a healthy relationship. There are ways that touch can be used skilfully, which are described in the Touch section.

All in all, this can be a difficult topic to face. Yet doing so can result in opportunities to strengthen relationships and for personal growth. If you are open to this approach, you may just find that your support network flourishes and provides you with what you need to continue shaping a positive future.

Encouragement points

- Family and friends can play a significant part in your journey onwards as you shape a positive future.
- There are practical ways they can help at the right time.
- They will need to understand your experiences and pain, so you can share your resources.
- Often people don't know how they can be helpful. You can guide them according to your needs.
- Many people value their independence and find it hard to ask for help. Yet this can be an important part of what you need to move forward.

Pacing

> *'Organising your activities, including recharge time, sets you up to move forward.'* RS

Pacing is a term that is commonly used in pain management, which is why I have included it here. However, I prefer to think about the way you plan, prioritise, and periodise your day, together with actively managing your energy—see the relevant sections.

The latter gives you more flexibility, allows for nuances, and takes into account the detail that is necessary to keep doing the basics as well as you can. Consistently doing the basics is what brings results as you are practising your skills and getting better at them.

Pacing or organising your day also sits closely with the art of setting your expectations. This is also an important section to read as you go about creating and curating your programme.

Encouragement points

See the following sections to become skilful at managing your day:

- Planning, prioritising, and periodising
- Energy
- Expectations

Sleep

'Everything's better when your sleep improves. It is a habit.' RS

Sleep is arguably one of the most important contributors to our sense of health and well-being. Most people know that just one night of disrupted sleep can cause a host of difficulties the next day. More pain, more anxiety, less resilience, and clarity of thought, all coming together as an unpleasant package. Of course, everyone will have days like this, meaning that different management strategies are needed.

Many people suffering from persistent pain have disturbed sleep. They may or may not have reported it, and if so, some have been given sleeping tablets. Such medication can induce a form of sleep, but it is not the same as natural sleep, making it perhaps a short-term option.

Over the past few years, much more has been learned about sleep. For example, the work of sleep scientist Matt Walker has done much to raise awareness with his book *Why We Sleep*, his TED talk, and his podcast. For a more in-depth look at sleep, I encourage you to check these out. As a consequence of this work and of others in the field, there are a number of practical things you can do based on research and understanding the importance of getting a good night's kip. Especially if you are trying to get the upper hand on your pain.

Overcoming pain is akin to learning. You are taking on board some new concepts and practising new skills. One of the key ingredients for learning is sleep. This is because memories are consolidated when we sleep, cementing what we have acquired during the day into something we can recall. A recent study showed that both non-REM and REM sleep are important (Tamaki et al., 2020), the former for the necessary neuroplasticity to improve performance and the latter for reducing plasticity to enable learning.

There are a lot of products on the market that claim to help. For instance, a range of pillows, supplements, diffusers, and others that aim to relax you. Some people may find that they help. Sedative medication is often prescribed by doctors. They can help people sleep, but this is not the same quality as natural sleep.

Before this though, there are practices, tools, and strategies that you can use, based on the knowledge that sleeping is a habit. Professor of sleep medicine at the University of Oxford, Colin Espie, talks about the five principles of good sleep health (2022): value, prioritise, personalise, trust, and protect. This is a good place to start. You can compare them to your current approach.

Five principles of good sleep

1. Value your sleep: you can choose to make it an important part of your life, a priority.
2. Prioritise sleep in your intentions and your actions.
3. Personalise your sleep habit: you need to discover what works for you in terms of pre-bed activities and timings (length of sleep, time for bed).
4. Trust: if you have created the conditions in the best way you can, then you can trust your sleep. Good sleepers expect to have good sleep, without thinking about it. You may have become very conscious of your sleep. Overthinking is a problem that typically worsens the situation.
5. Protect your sleep: try to keep the timings consistent, do what you can to be calm on your way to bed, think about your lifestyle and dietary choices, and create an environment conducive to sleep.

This is a good framework. Let's now look at some practices you can implement to use it.

You can create the conditions for sleep not only in how you prepare for bed but also in how you manage your energy and lifestyle day to day.

Interviewed for a Washington Post article, the director of the Yale Paediatric Sleep Centre, Craig Canapari said: 'It is really important to have reasonable expectations about sleep and also realising that you can only set the table for sleep. You can invite it to come, but you can't control when it happens.' As ever, we must try to focus on what we can control rather than what we can't. As it is with pain, expectations play a significant role. It is considered normal to have the occasional disturbed night. Knowing this means you will not be surprised when you do, and you may have an insight into why.

Managing your day

Sleep at night is in part related to how you manage your whole day and hence reflects lifestyle. The hour or so before bed will be addressed below, but it goes beyond this as you try to build your sleep drive over the day. There is an accumulation of the chemical adenosine in your brain, responsible for the feeling of sleepiness that motivates you to go to bed (Sims et al., 2013).

Actively managing your energy means that you have regular recharge and rest breaks when necessary throughout the day (see Energy, Pacing, and Planning sections). These can be at certain times and after a time chunk when you have been doing some work or an exercise, allowing your body to adapt to what you have done, returning to a balanced state.

People often describe how they feel groggy and tired in the morning, unrested, and as if they have not really slept. In this case, having a morning routine (see Morning routine section) becomes more important—a way to get yourself going, even a little. You are trying to create a sleep habit, which means you go to bed and get up at the same time each day.

Designing your day, you have your recharge points. Here you choose a practice that lifts your energy. Some find it useful to make a list of things that give positive energy. For example, movement, fresh air, a cold shower, a hug, talking to someone, and listening to music. It will be personal of course. Together with using your chosen energiser, you can practise being present to notice how it feels, marking your change in state with awareness. Bringing yourself to the here and now is important because it is only by being present that we can address our own suffering. If we are somewhere else in our mind, we can't.

Setting your timings

We are aiming for seven and a half to eight hours of restful sleep according to sleep science—the ideal. However, this is not a realistic starting point for many, especially if you are suffering pain. There is a skill in setting goals, as they need to feel reachable in the future. Becoming over-focused on the goals can be a problem as you lose touch with what you need to do at this moment. If this happens, you are focusing on the prize over the process. You will need to switch that around and focus on the process: what is my best step now?

Initially you may be thinking that you will do your best to create a sleep habit, sowing the seeds for better rest. You can, as you know, only create the conditions and trust that your body will respond as you gradually shift your expectations towards sleeping better.

When you are setting your new bedtime, it typically works better if you nudge the time. For example, if you have been going to bed at 1 am, you start your new routine at 1230 or 1245am, become used to this, and then nudge again. This makes it more realistic and brings expectations and reality in closer alignment.

Light

When you wake up, try to absorb yourself in natural light. Open the curtains, let the sunlight in (challenging in some places!), or whatever light the day is offering. Daylight plays a key role in our body clock regulation, turning off the effects of melatonin, which tells us it is night-time.

Twenty minutes of light in the morning will get you started. Try to build this into your routine, avoiding dark rooms or coffee shops if you can. Angle everything, all your intent, towards 'its daytime'.

In the evening, darkness infers that it is time to start getting sleepy. Create a cool, dark environment for your bedroom that is conducive to sleep.

Eating and drinking

What and when you eat can affect your sleep. Whilst it goes beyond the scope of this book to discuss diet in detail, there are certain principles you can follow.

Try to avoid heavy meals late at night. In fact, any food eaten later in the evening will create a greater demand as the gut moves into idling according to the circadian rhythm. Attempting to digest food at this time will almost certainly disrupt your sleep habit. This being the case, you may decide to eat your evening meal before 8pm.

Coffee is very popular. People enjoy the taste and the culture. It is also used to bring alertness, which is fine depending on the time of day. Caffeine in your coffee stops the effect of adenosine, the chemical that builds during the day to create the feeling of sleepiness, and hence wakes you up. The problem that people can have is that a quarter of the caffeine will still be in the brain twelve hours later. So, if you have a coffee at 2 pm or 3 pm, in the early hours of the morning you have a chemical in your system that is all about being awake at the time when you need to be asleep.

Some people will claim that they can sleep despite a late coffee after dinner. Indeed, they do fall asleep; however, we know that this affects deep sleep, so they will not be getting the same refreshment.

Even less popular is the truth about alcohol. Just one drink will disrupt your sleep. There is a belief that a tipple before bed can help fall asleep. Matt Walker is clear on this: 'Many people see alcohol as a sleep aid. Unfortunately, it's one of the greatest misunderstood substances when it comes to sleep. It is not a sleep aid at all.'

REM sleep is disturbed by alcohol. During this phase of sleep, memories and learning take place, meaning that alcohol disrupts these important processes. Just one glass is enough.

So whilst you may believe that your glass of wine helps you relax and get off to sleep, it is actually impacting the quality.

Exercise

It is known that exercise helps both getting off to sleep and staying asleep. Of course, the problem of pain includes being less active, meaning that there is less contribution to the building sleep drive over the day. Being able to gradually increase activity levels will help achieve better rest at night together with the slew of other benefits, but also working on a better sleep habit increases the likelihood of exercising. It seems that there could be a relationship going in both directions, giving more possibilities (Kline, 2014).

Better mood, less anxiety, greater fitness and strength, improved concentration and memory all come in the wake of regular exercise. In turn, these are helpful for sleep. For instance, if your anxiety levels are lowered by exercising, then this will reduce the impact of worry on your sleep.

One of the important themes of getting better is building wellness. Exercise and activity come under this banner within your daily programme (see Exercise and Building health sections).

Naps

According to Walker (2021), if you are finding getting to sleep or staying asleep difficult, you should avoid naps. This is because they release the pressure of the sleep drive that is otherwise building through the day towards the feelings of sleepiness before bed. The nap in this case is encouraging a state of wakefulness when you want to settle down for the night.

Evening routine

You have now decided what time you will go to bed because sleep is a valued part of your day and the way you self-care. How do you organise your evening to work with your sleep drive so that you are ready for sleep when the time comes?

Due to past experiences, we tend to have expectations about going to bed. Some people tell themselves that another bad night is on the way, or abandon any routine because it makes no difference. Changing our thinking is a vital first step. Where can we put our attention? One place is upon our efforts and intent. So, process over prize, as we set the conditions for better sleep to come. Or, sowing seeds. Whichever analogy, it is important to remember several things:

1. You can only create the best conditions by choosing to do certain things
2. It takes time for a consistent sleep habit to bear fruit; probably months
3. There will be ups and downs

But if you keep going, doing the basics well, there will be improvements.

You can control the following in most cases:

1. What you expose yourself to in the evening: for instance, the programmes or films you watch, the podcasts you listen to, the books you read. As you head towards bed time, if you want to induce sleep, then the content needs to be calming.
2. When you eat.
3. Your last drink choice: for example, a herbal tea, water (rather than alcohol or coffee).
4. When you stop using your device. Ideally an hour before bed as the light affects melatonin levels and shifts the body clock some three hours. There is also a chance that the content is rousing, for instance, an action-packed movie, something upsetting or thought-provoking. One could argue that even watching the news at 10 pm is a way to disrupt sleep on that basis.
5. Your narrative. Firstly, you notice what you are telling yourself about sleeping. For example, are you anticipating another bad night, hopeful of a good night or perhaps not much in the way of thinking beforehand. Either way, there is an implicit expectation of what is to come based on past experiences, even if you are not overtly thinking about it. Secondly, you can create a new narrative based on realistic expectations. By this I mean that instead of saying to yourself, I will sleep well, you say, I will do my best to create the conditions for sleep. Some people then find it

useful to combine this with imagery. When thinking about going to bed, you are imagining yourself comfy and asleep in bed. This way you are pointing your resources towards what you want to achieve.

Essentially you have choices.

Why is it important to you? Remind yourself that it is because you value your sleep and your health. What is the cost of not improving your sleep habit? Think in a year or five years. Then think about how it would be to have better sleep. What difference would that make to your life?

The question you can ask yourself is: does this make it more likely or less likely to help me sleep? The answer will give you a guide.

Encouragement points

- Sleep is a vital part of recovery and overcoming pain.
- A sleep habit is about bedtime and how you manage your energy throughout the day.
- Sleep is a habit that must be grooved over an extended period of time—there is no quick fix.
- You create the conditions with the choices you make—this you can control.
- Design your routine for bedtime that encourages sleepiness at least an hour before bed.

Social media

'How you use social media determines whether it is helpful or a hindrance.' RS

Social media is a source of useful and not so useful information. With billions of users worldwide, many people suffering from persistent pain use different platforms to try and find out more about their experiences. They may also be looking for validation and to become part of a group. Again, some are positive, and some less so.

You may have already ventured into the online world, including search engines, and made some discoveries. There are plenty of sites, blogs, and opinions. How do you decide what is good quality information and advice?

Below I share some tips on how to get the best out of social media. But there is another consideration. When do you look?

Many people tell me that they check their phones before bed, in bed, and during the middle of the night. As with any action, there are pluses and minuses. The pluses include relieving that sense of needing to check a device and finding an explanation for a worry or question you have. The minuses are the ongoing compulsion to look at your phone (habit), waking yourself up before bed or when you are needing sleep and the quality of judgement when reading a page, post, or tweet.

Further, reading something that triggers a stress response will also affect your ability to sleep. This will potentially set you off down a route of worry and concern that keeps you up and awake.

If you are going to look at social media and the internet, which most people will, there are some principles that you can follow.

When and how long

You can set the times when you will do some research, thinking about the best time of day to be able to choose reliable sources and absorb the information. This may also include how long you spend online. Many people have difficulty concentrating, so chunking your time, just as you do with other activities, can be a useful method.

For some people, it can be tempting to check devices and look at social media at night if you wake up.

Check your sources

Establishing who the article is written by and for helps you understand any biases and agendas that are being pushed.

For pain, the NHS, the British Pain Society, the Physiotherapy Pain Association, PubMed, and the International Association for the Study of Pain are good places to start. However, no source is foolproof, so there is no absolute guarantee of quality or accuracy. You may like to discuss any findings you make with your healthcare provider to make sense of it, or to understand whether it is relevant to you.

There is no silver bullet

I am typically suspicious of miracle cures and quick fixes. The science of pain to date tells us that this is not what happens, as much as we would like it to be the case. There have been occasions when the mass media has jumped on a story based on a study that has shown certain results. We need to be very careful about how the results are reported. Much research is done on rodents, so we cannot immediately assume the same in humans. We must also check the study methodology carefully.

The bottom line is that to overcome a pain problem, meaning that pain is not the dominant force in your life that it has been, or that it has resolved, depending on your circumstances, takes understanding, self-care, and practice.

Interpreting statistics

Most people do not have training in how to interpret statistics. This can pose a problem because the headlines steal the show. Digging deeper, you can discover that the number of subjects in the study was small, or that there was no comparison group. This has a serious implication for the results and conclusions.

The gold standard for research studies is randomised controlled trials (RCTs) when different groups are compared, including a control group that receives no treatment. This method allows the researchers to elucidate the active components of a particular treatment and how effective it is for a condition.

There are always limitations with studies, and these are normally outlined clearly in the paper.

Other people's stories

When we read about other people, we can take this as our truth. Of course, this is not the case, but it can feel like it when we become bound up in their narrative. Many people who are suffering share their stories. This gives us important insights and helps us to understand their lived experience. However, it is unique to them and does not mean you will suffer the same outcomes.

Some people choose to look out for encouraging stories. Again, these are not your outcomes, but you may gain some helpful ideas based on what they have done.

Caution applies here with treatments that people have tried and then recommend. It is great to hear that someone has found benefit, but you need to understand if this applies to you and weigh up any risks and the costs. There are some enormously expensive treatments and programmes being offered in different places around the world.

My suggestion is that if you find something that appears to be a good prospect, look for the evidence and a scientific explanation. You can also ask about the success rates and risks.

Influencers

There are people on social media with many followers. This does not mean that their advice is necessarily correct or relevant to you.

As a distraction

It is understandable that people use social media to distract themselves from their pain. To immerse in the images and videos can be compelling and gratifying. A new word was coined to describe this particular action: doom-scrolling.

Whilst it can feel good, and perhaps unrealistic to say that we won't do it, there are consequences. Evidence suggests that spending more time on a digital device and on social media are both linked with anxiety and depression (Ghaemi, 2020; Vannucci et al., 2017). The timing of use can be relevant, for instance, teens using social media at night predicted poorer sleep in one study (Woods et al., 2016). When sleep is affected, this has the knock-on impact for mood, anxiety, and pain as well as general energy levels.

We do have a need to know, which can explain why it feels right to scroll. Fear of missing out (FOMO), keeping up to date so that you are in the discussion, and trying to allay concerns about the world are all reasons. Some of this is within our natural instinct that evolved to keep us in the group. It was important to have this status to survive when we were cave dwellers. To be outed usually meant death. This is thought to be the reason for the power of shame, which is to feel that you are excluded from the group (Steindl, 2020).

You may be amused by memes, entertained by videos, but also triggered by other content. You are a thinking, feeling human being, and whatever you expose yourself to will be impacting upon you. Do you find yourself getting upset because other people's feeds are showing that they have a great life? Of course, all feeds are curated by the person and some only want to show a certain perspective on their life.

The seeds you water will grow. Gathering insights into what is shaping you, including social media, puts you in a position of understanding to enable you to make the best choices.

If there is a strong urge to check your channels, and with a short-term reward of pain relief, it can be hard to stop or limit. It seems understandable that there can be an addictive element, as you seek to meet your needs. Yet the flip side of possible increased feelings of anxiety and depression should be considered seriously. Conscious awareness of the pluses and minuses puts you in a position of making the best choice in line with your picture of success.

Encouragement points

- Social media is part of many people's lives, but how do you use it?
- Find reliable sources of information.
- Remember that someone else's story is not yours.
- Plan how much time you spend (roughly), put limits on your device and think about the time of day.
- Make a conscious choice based on the pluses and minuses—there are risks for your health despite how it feels.
- Is social media helping you achieve your goals?

Challenging moments

'Challenging moments can become learning opportunities.' RS

You have probably realised through your own experiences that your journey is up and down. That is the reality because life is up and down. Regardless of your preferences, life happens. I have addressed this in different sections of the book, in particular setting your expectations in line with reality.

If there is a mismatch, for instance, believing that recovery is a straight line, then you will feel like you are not doing very well. Instead, when you know there are going to be challenges but you have ways to meet them skilfully to keep moving forward, your confidence builds.

Knowing and accepting that there will be challenging moments means that you can prepare by developing certain skills. You can also have the intention to deal with them in the best way that you can. One of the overarching principles of this book and my way is to highlight that you are always doing your best, even if it doesn't turn out the way you want.

And by the way, when this happens (it will—plenty!), you may think you made a 'bad' decision. Not necessarily true. Not getting the outcome you want does not make the decision a bad one. It was the best decision you could have made at that moment (it is easy to look back and think something different …). The key question is, what can I learn?

So how can you best meet such moments? The practices and skills in this section will add to your existing resources. You may well already have some ways of doing this successfully. The question to ask yourself is whether they are helpful? Are they delivering the results that you want?

One of the main themes to overcome pain is by living life. This is in the choices you make and how you live moment to moment. The bulk of your time is made up of this, with far less time being dedicated to daily practices to achieve your goals and the skills of being well. All are important of course.

You may be thinking that you are really trying to live your life, yet still have pain and limitations. Remember that this is a process and where you are now is not where you will be when you seek to follow a path towards your pictures of success. Keep them in mind, but know where you are now and the direction you are heading.

Living life means you are connecting with what matters and engaging or re-engaging with valued activities and people. In doing this you will be in different and better states, both biological and experiential. How do you feel when you think of a loved one? Or a situation that was funny or uplifting? Take a moment now to close your eyes and bring this to mind. What happens in your body? You may notice the shift, even subtle. This can grow. It is a skill to practise so that you get better at changing gears, or states when you need and want.

The way you meet each moment and situation determines what it is like for you. It is not what is happening but how you relate to it that matters, is a key insight. I encourage you to reread the last sentence. Why? Because how you relate to it makes it what it is for you, and determines if you are then in a resourceful state or not. The way you think of what is happening needs to open up possibilities for action that take you in the direction of your picture of success. What can you learn? How can you respond with skill rather than react?

Commonly people react to difficult moments and situations. These are often automatic and learned thoughts, feelings, and actions. Again, the question is whether these reactions are helpful or not? When there is little or no space between what happens and your reaction, no choices exist. Learning to create space to make the best decision is a more skilful and measured way to respond. Less reactive, more responsive.

One of the day-to-day practices that help you be more skilful is meditation because you become more present more often. When you are present, or 'awake', you see things more clearly because you have built your ability to be aware. It is the awareness that starts to change things for the better. It is the awareness that allows you to heal.

To be aware of your thoughts is very different from being entangled with your thoughts. Rather than being blown around by the winds of your preferences or automatic reactions, you have the clarity and calmness to understand and meet your own needs. There is a big difference between feeling certain emotions such as anger and fear and being mindful of them.

They come, they go. Nothing is permanent as you begin to see and understand in the way you live. You learn not to identify with such feeling states and instead know that they will pass by.

In the following pages are practices you can try. The proof is in the pudding, as I always say. Try to notice your experiences. What is it like when you use these tools as different ways to meet or respond to challenging moments? Some people find it useful to write down what works in their journal. I certainly encourage studying your own successes.

Apply the brakes

One of the first steps is to slow things down. Feelings and thoughts seem to be gathering momentum, and you want to bring some control and clarity. To do this, you can apply the brakes. How?

Breathe.

Taking 2–3 breaths, slow if you can, brings some presence and awareness to the moment. It also changes your state, moving from being largely sympathetic (fright, flight, freeze) to more parasympathetic (restorative, calming).

Even a slight slowing of momentum can give you the opportunity to see things as they are, rather than being caught up. With some space and clarity, you can make your next best decision, which could be more breathing, perhaps moving or something else that is calming and soothing. You can also reflect on what happened so that in the future, you understand the trigger and respond differently. You don't have to do things the same way, especially if the result of your reactions is more suffering.

When you learn to drive or ski or cycle, one of the first skills you learn is how to slow down and stop. It is easy to accelerate, but reigning yourself in is trickier. How quickly do you get angry? How long does it take to calm down?

Practicing breathing throughout the day helps develop both the skill and the awareness that you can use it. Initially, it may not occur to you to use breathing, but gradually it becomes a way of calming. In some cases, you may find movement is also needed to help you change state together with the breath.

Movement

You have probably noticed how you feel differently when you get up and move around. There is a quick change of state that starts to happen even before you move. In anticipation, your brain predicts standing up and organises the relevant energy systems and diverts blood flow. Your blood pressure increases in preparation so that by the time you are on your feet, there is enough oxygen in your brain to continue what you are doing. If your blood pressure does not go up, when you stand, you can feel lightheaded or dizzy.

For many years, when a writer has become stuck with writer's block, the suggestion has been to walk around the block. It seems that many discoveries have been made whilst the person is strolling along. Science shows that walking increases blood flow to the brain with each step. This would be expected to change how you feel compared to being sedentary.

There are many ways to move all the parts of your body. Endless exercises in all manner of positions offer opportunities for most circumstances. Sometimes a gentle rocking, other times a stretch, change of position, or a walk. For most people I work with, these movements are encouraged to be within their window of tolerance (for more see section Movement). In other words, have a good experience of movement. There is an importance because what you do now in this moment is shaping your expectations for the next time.

Finding ways to move, perhaps with some guidance, that change your state becomes an important part of your day-to-day toolbox. In time, you may update or progress them. What you are doing now to get better, will not necessarily be what you are doing in time to come. They serve a purpose for now.

Reframing

There is a narrative you are telling yourself about what is happening. Thoughts and memories contribute as does the feeling of your body—they all come together as one lived experience. Ethan Kross calls this chatter (Kross, 2022). Others rumination. Whatever you name it, when you listen, it is utterly convincing (Brown, 2019).

Realising that these are just thoughts and that they may not bear any relation to what is actually happening is a powerful shift in perspective. Putting forward an alternative that is closer to the truth of the present moment can wind down the strong emotions. Of course, this requires self-awareness and presence, which as you know are developed in mindful practice.

Kross suggests some ways of doing this in his book *Chatter* (2021). Essentially, we cannot stop our thoughts and neither should we try. Like King Canute, you cannot prevent the tide for coming in as much as halting thoughts arising. Instead, we recognise their appearance and disappearance. They always pass by, although can recur as you know well.

1. Distance yourself from the thought: (a) what would you say to a friend who asked for your advice? (b) use your name; _____ (your name) is thinking (c) say the word 'thoughts' when you notice them. Some people describe a change in quality of their experience. An awakening, a presence or something else. This is an insight into your own self-awareness when you become aware of your thoughts and the chatter, rather than being caught up in it and suffering.

2. How would you speak to a friend? What advice would you give to them (when invited)? This again is a form of distancing, allowing you to try and look at the situation more objectively. If there is a tendency to speak to yourself in a critical way, or even unkindly, you will notice a different tone that you use with someone else who you care about. Naturally in time and with practice, you are aiming to speak to yourself with more compassion. This is one way to see how through your own repositioning.

3. Use your name: there are several ways you can bring presence and awareness to the moment, rather than being caught up. Saying your name to yourself is one. So in my case, I say to myself: Richmond is thinking. It can sound a little strange, but when you practise and notice the feel of what it is like on saying this to yourself. You realise that you have pulled back and created some space to see what is really happening.

4. Say 'Thoughts': this is the second way of breaking the train of thoughts, similar to (3) when you create space to see.

5. Several other practices that people can find useful are to think about how you will feel about the situation in a month or a year's time and to reinterpret the feelings in your body. Again, both put some distance between the sense of yourself as a thinker and the thoughts. It is when

you become caught up in the thoughts and the stories that suffering increases.

Rethinking the feelings in your body helps to change what they are like for you. Recall that our perceptions are shaped in part by our thinking and beliefs. This means that we can shift our perspective to change our experience. That is not to say that we can always think our way out of feeling certain ways or pain. But changing the way we look at things creates an opportunity for different ways of responding and having a more hopeful outlook. Both of these are important for moving onwards in a better direction.

You also know now that our thinking is embodied. This means that when we think differently, our actions and perceptions change. It also means that moving or taking different actions will change your thinking. Perception, action, and thinking all come together. This presents many opportunities once understood, forming the basis of many of the tools and practices you are learning in this book.

For example, you may feel butterflies in your stomach—a common feeling. When you feel it, what do you tell yourself about the cause? Some people will interpret this as meaning you are anxious. Others will tell themselves that they are excited. It will depend on past learning and experiences together with the context you are in that moment. What happens when you find yourself entangled in the story of being anxious, but then you change it to being excited? How does it feel now?

It is not just about the feeling. It's about what that is like, how it is embodied, and the interwoven story. They come together to make it what it is. There is no separation. You realise this when you examine your own experience.

RAIN

RAIN stands for recognise, allow, investigate, and nurture. It can appear to be a step-wise approach, but with practice it becomes more seamless.

A proponent of RAIN is Tara Brach, a well-known meditation teacher and psychotherapist. Tara describes RAIN as a mindful and compassionate practice, which is a perfect combination for moments of suffering.

From her website, Tara summarises the steps (https://www.tarabrach.com/rain):

Recognise what is happening;
Allow the experience to be there, just as it is;

Investigate with interest and care;
Nurture with self-compassion.

In the modern world you often are encouraged to avoid pain and difficulties, or to cover them up, or to somehow distract yourself and turn the other way. Whilst in the short term you can feel better, and even rewarded (by avoiding pain), this is not the route to transformation. Like squeezing a long balloon at one end, it will pop out somewhere else.

It takes courage and understanding to turn towards your suffering. But this is the way of transforming your experiences. RAIN helps you by giving you a framework until it becomes a natural way. Not only is this a way forward, but is a practice that you become better at using at different times in your life. Pain is not the only challenge.

Recognise: some people find it helpful to name what is happening. For example, there is pain. In taking this step you are creating space to think rather than becoming embroiled in the thinking about what you are feeling. This is in contrast to avoidance or trying to cover up the pain. You are turning towards your lived experience in that moment with the intent of responding skilfully and compassionately.

You can add labelling (see below), which is when you use an adjective to describe what is happening, creating space to see what is actually happening. There is often a shift in the feel when you label. For example, 'Thinking, thinking, thinking', 'There is pain', or 'There is tension'. This is a skill you can use stand-alone through the day to pull back and bring awareness to the situation.

Allow: again this takes courage to be with the pain without trying to do anything aside from be present. You are not trying to change anything, understanding that this lived experience is the best explanation for your circumstances at this moment (biology, environment, context).

Investigate: in a kindly way, you consider your circumstances—what is going on for you right now? This insight is strengthened with regular meditation practice and is invaluable for understanding oneself and the way you think. In doing so, you create space to make your best decisions, always considering the circumstances. You might think about where you are, what you are doing, what you have been doing, who you are with, what is on your mind, any memories floating by, and what it is you are about to do.

Nurture: this is when you take some kind of compassionate action to self soothe, reassure yourself, and change state. This is in line with your picture of success. Once you are feeling better and clearer, you can then make your next best decision, aiming to reconnect with what matters—a value-based decision. You may simply resume what you were doing, having self-soothed, and reassured yourself that you are ok. This way you are addressing that part of you that is suffering and concerned, rather than ignoring or dismissing.

Initially RAIN can feel like a step-wise practice. In time, it becomes more seamless.

Like all the practices and tools in the book, the more you use them, the more skilled you become. Some will work better than others, so you can focus on those that deliver the results you want.

Labelling

Labelling can be used stand-alone or as part of one of the other practices. For example, during RAIN when recognising and acknowledging what is happening. You might say to yourself: 'there is pain', or 'there is tension'.

By labelling the raw experience, you give yourself distance between you (subject) and what you are feeling (object). In a sense you can look at it and see it for what it is. A passing experience that is being generated top down by your body systems is the best guess to explain your current circumstances, based on prior history.

Within the space you can choose how to relate and respond to the experience. Beyond labelling, you can ask yourself if the experience is a good explanation? Is your reality a good take on the reality of life?

Perhaps you are feeling pain in your back whilst sitting in a chair. Is this activity a real threat to your integrity? Is there actual danger? No, of course not. Except you may believe that there is if you have been given an explanation for your pain that includes something about squashing discs or nerves. But now you know that this is not how pain works.

Plenty of people 'squash' their tissues without pain. So, there must be more to it. Essentially knowing that you are safe goes some way to creating a calm perspective so that you can decide what to do next. What is my best course of action?

You have labelled the pain: there is pain. You have investigated what is happening, including whether your thoughts and stories are accurate and helpful. Now you are clear to take action. Now, just because you know you are not doing any harm, it doesn't mean you have to sit there and suffer! There is a need behind the pain experience.

It is going to be sensible to move and improve your experience of sitting. After all, as you know, getting better requires that you create evidence of getting better. You are curating and creating better experiences of sitting in this case and building the time that you can do so within your window of tolerance.

You can also label thoughts: 'thinking, thinking, thinking'; if you have a tendency to ruminate and get caught up in your stories. Again, this pulls you back and allows you the opportunity to ask yourself: is this thought helpful? And to recognise that it is just a thought.

Regular practices

Some of these practices are ones you can develop outside of the tricky times, thereby raising your skill level for when you need them. For example, breathing awareness, RAIN, mindfulness can all be part of a day-to-day routine. They create the conditions for calm and clarity as you go about your life, and then form a way of dealing with the inevitable bumps in the road. The less the disturbance to the inner world, the clearer you will be to make your next best choice.

As I have said elsewhere, in Western society we are not taught how to suffer. It seems like an alien concept, yet with suffering being a part of life, surely we are missing a trick? To wait until it is already really difficult makes it much harder.

Encouragement points

- There will inevitably be challenging moments, ups and downs. Accepting this as the way is important.
- Having skills and practices you can use will help you respond more effectively.
- When faced with a difficult or painful time, this can become an opportunity to see how you are transforming your suffering.
- Challenging moments are an opportunity to get back on track.
- They will pass. Nothing is permanent.

Moment to moment

'Moment to moment decisions govern the quality of your life to an extent, so awareness, clarity and presence matter.' RS

The bulk of the day is taken up with you living your life in the best way you can. Remember that you could do it no better with the circumstances as they were. At all times, you are doing your best. This is not an excuse by the way. It is a reality that can be combined with taking responsibility and seeking to shape a positive future.

Your practices, exercises, and tools only take up a small portion of your day. How long do you spend on them in total? An hour? Then there is the rest of the time. How do you handle the remainder of the day? How are you meeting and relating to the moment to moment? The quality of these decisions and your current habits of thought and action are having a huge bearing on your quality of life.

Chronic pain is a complex process that emerges from your entire life rather than a discrete, isolated experience. Whether and how you feel pain is influenced by many factors that have been before and that exist at the moment, as you now know. And how you meet each moment is determined by how you are and the skills available to you. This is dynamic. If you are feeling stressed and overwhelmed, fewer possibilities will exist because your mind closes down in this state. If you can remain balanced and calm, more options will be available, particularly if you have been practising certain skills.

A firefighter does not become immediately skilled at being calm in the face of a furnace. Firefighters learn ways to deal with themselves and situations in the classroom and then in mock scenarios that gradually become more challenging as they progress and grow. It is the same for you, developing your skills by practising in a safer, easier environment, so that when you need to use them, you do so with greater effect. Each time you do this, especially as you go about your day-to-day activities, you get a little more experienced and better for the next time, and so on.

Ways that you can meet arising moments litter this book. You may be able to think of some now, perhaps those you are using. As ever, awareness and presence play a large role in this, together with existing habits. The way you habitually approach life determines the quality of your life. Habits happen automatically, but you can still be aware of what is happening. Building awareness then, is important. How do you do this?

One of the common ways of becoming more aware and present is to meditate as you know now (see this section). Having a daily sitting practice builds your awareness, which is the first step to healing—healing referring to transforming and easing your suffering. There is a huge difference between being aware of what is happening, how you are feeling, what you are thinking and being caught up in them; the autopilot. You could call it being awake versus sleepwalking through your life.

Being awake means that you are open and accepting of what is happening in this moment—the only moment. Due to your preferences, you may resist what is happening because you don't like it. Understandable. But unfortunately, whether you like it or not makes no difference to what is already happening. What resistance does is make the coming moments worse.

Suffering comes from wanting to be somewhere else or for the circumstances to be different to how they are. As soon as you see this, you can practice dropping back into awareness of what is happening, cultivating an impartial mind that is open, connected, and non-reactive. This is meeting a moment with skill and poise to create space for options. You neither push away what you don't want nor hold onto what you do want. Instead, you notice the comings and goings, for if experiences such as pain can arise, they can also pass by.

Encouragement points

- Whilst there are important practices, exercises, and tools to work on each day, the bulk of your time is the day to day. Which practices will you use to meet these moments skilfully so that you are in a resourceful state?
- Being open to whatever arises and letting it pass by instead of pushing away or holding on eases suffering. Your daily practices help you achieve this as you live your life; skills 'on the go'.
- What you practise you will get better at (as long as your practice is high quality and prioritised).
- Your daily habits and choices contribute significantly to your quality of life. Which will you practice and hone on a route of mastery?

Acceptance

'Acceptance is not giving in. It is simply acknowledging what is actually happening and starting there.' RS

The 'A' word: Acceptance

You may have heard it or have had it suggested as a way to move forward. The opposite is to resist and fight your situation. Whilst it is understandable and often encouraged (in society), this latter approach is a cause of more suffering. The battle-type language is often used to describe what the person must do to win or overcome their condition. However, this has been questioned in recent times.

Oncologist Shikha Jain recently wrote on the matter in relation to fighting cancer (2020): 'This type of rhetoric can be damaging to patients, their families and their caregivers. If a patient sees cancer treatment as a battle that must be fought, they can feel they have not done enough if the treatment does not work, or if they cannot tolerate the side effects of treatment.'

Some people maybe spurred on, of course, but others may feel they have to pretend that they are fighting or fear being open about their struggle. This heaps on pressure to be and act a certain way, adding to the stress.

Writing in the Guardian, journalist Ian Sample reported on a study by Hauser (2019) that examined the effects of using battle language for cancer. He wrote:

Framing cancer in military terms made treatment seem more difficult and left people feeling more fatalistic about the illness, believing there was little they could do to reduce their risk, researchers found ... And while the language is intended to motivate people and make them more vigilant at spotting symptoms and getting them examined, the study found no evidence this was the case.

What has this to do with pain? Some people use this kind of language: I am fighting the pain, or I won't give into this pain, or I will beat this pain. To take this approach implies that there is a war going on within you. Now consider what a battlefield looks like and the kind of things that are implied, when you are actually trying to ease your suffering and bring calmness and healing in order to improve your life.

Further, if you are thinking about fighting, who are you fighting? Or what are you fighting? The pain you may say. But the pain is emerging from you, the person, so again you fight yourself. This can be hard to hear or read, because if you are not battling the pain, you may think you are giving up. You are not. That is a big misunderstanding.

You have not given up. Acceptance does not mean surrendering (war language again) or giving into the pain. Instead, it is an acknowledgment of your current situation and circumstances. It is impossible to move forward without this vital insight. Resistance stops you progressing. One of the reasons is that the energy you put into the fight means there is less to put into improving your life. You find yourself focusing on the pain rather than what it is you want to achieve.

Many people say at the beginning that they want to achieve pain relief. I understand. But in practice, by focusing on the pain, you will do the opposite. This sounds paradoxical. However, as you deepen your understanding of your pain, it will make sense to you. If it doesn't, then I recommend that you review the 'What is pain?' section. You'll know that you need to do this if you are finding this particularly hard to take on board. You are certainly not alone in finding this is a sticky subject though. Some people will need to address this in therapy sessions in order to refocus on a forward path.

The more you focus on the pain and trying to treat it, the worse the outcome. The more you focus on the way you want to live, build wellness, and manage the difficult times (i.e. painful), the better the outcome. Just treating the pain keeps your attention on it, which usually makes it worse, and the effects will only ever be short-term. Whereas creating better and good experiences (states) helps you to create flexibility in the systems that are generating your perceptions; in other words, getting unstuck. They have become stuck by repeated episodes of pain that result in an ongoing (subconscious) expectation of pain, even when there is no actual threat. You may have been doing worse than expected—you expected to get better but then did not. Now you need to match expectations with reality (see Expectations) to start moving in a better direction.

To do this, you need to be able to accept where you are right now. To say to yourself, here I am and this is my starting point. I accept that I have pain in all these different circumstances, and this is what I am going to do to move forward. Dropping the resistance can make all the difference. Many people have described this transformational shift in perspective to me and how it has helped them to put their efforts into getting better. It is hard without doubt, some days it is easier than others, but it is possible and you have the courage to do it.

As I said above, many people need help with this step. If you are finding it too difficult alone, then I encourage you to reach out.

Encouragement points

- Acceptance is not giving in.
- Acceptance is to acknowledge your circumstances as they are right now so that you can make the best decisions based on what matters.
- Acceptance is not weakness. Instead, it is the strength to be present with your situation and suffering to transform your experience.

Habits

> 'Each time you repeat a thought or action, it is a practice for the future. Habits matter, either taking you toward your picture of success or away.' RS

Much of the work for overcoming pain is about forming new habits. The habits that we have, it could be said, influence the quality of our lives. They are the things we do over and over, often without thought, that create the conditions for how we are. There is a lag of course. The things I am doing today will not manifest for some time. This is one of the reasons why starting to exercise is challenging. Although you may feel satisfaction having been for a walk or to the gym (plus aches and pains of course), you will not see or feel any changes with regards to your body or fitness. That will come months later, but only if you stick to a routine. Pay day is not everyday!

So how do we keep going when there is no obvious or immediate reward? So much in life is immediate now. Clothes, take-aways, books, electronics, and many other material goods can be ordered and arrive that day or soon afterwards. But the important stuff, health, a career, and relationships, all take time and effort and practice over and over. Small incremental steps, often with plateaus when nothing seems to change, are the way. There are no hacks or short cuts or quick fixes.

The same is true for pain—no quick fixes.

Instead, day-to-day practice of certain skills and exercises plus better and better ways of dealing with difficult moments and feelings. This emphasises the importance of your existing habits and forming new ones as needed, in order to achieve your picture of success. Here are some questions to consider.

What does your picture of success look like? What kinds of habits do you need in order to be successful? What would that version of you be doing each day?

Habits of thought and action

Habits are not just the things you do. They form the way you think about yourself and the world. Part of this is in the way that you speak.

Thich Nhat Hanh wrote a wonderful book entitled The Art of Communicating (2013) that addresses this fundamental part of life and our health. Thinking about how you speak to yourself, to others, and about others is revealing in how we see the world. For instance, getting caught up in gossip or talking about someone unkindly when they are not there presents you in a particular light. Instead, coming through a compassionate lens means that you see things for what they really are and understand human suffering, wanting to help rather than add more fuel to the fire. This is known as Right Speech in Buddhism.

You can discover in yourself the typical tone you take in your inner dialogue by taking a moment to reflect. Do you encourage yourself? Do you look for the positives? This dialogue is shaping your experiences and what you see, so is of vital importance. It will also have an impact on your actions. They are inextricably tied together. This is why changing your narrative changes the world you perceive.

Forming a habit

There are some principles you can follow to create a new habit. It starts with thinking about the person you want to be so that you can make decisions accordingly; stepping into those shoes. One simple way of doing this is to come up with three words that describe that version of you and remind yourself of them through the day. If you can, add some imagery so you see yourself in that way and then step into those shoes.

   1. Think about the person you want to be

'Be the change you want to see in the world' are the words often misattributed to Gandhi. However, they remain useful words because they demonstrate how we mirror the world, which is what he did actually say. Gandhi stated, 'If we could change ourselves, the tendencies in the world would also change. As man changes his own nature, so does the attitude of the world change towards him … A wonderful thing it is and the source of our happiness. We need not wait to see what others do.'

This is a very practical insight and potentially transformational. You can practise immediately and notice what it is like. Firstly, check in on your current attitude towards life. How do you feel? In this mode and mood, how does the world appear to you? Now close your eyes and think about someone or something you love. Let the image appear, even if grainy or perhaps unclear. The intent is enough. Notice how you feel when you focus on this; does anything change in you? Remember that what you focus on governs how you feel. By shifting your focus, you are changing state. Once you have spent a few moments practising, now notice how the world appears to you.

This is a basic insight from different philosophical traditions, but not one we have necessarily been introduced to before. It may seem strange therefore, but I hope with practice, you will develop a sense of how changing your state and inner being, changes the way the world is towards you. A further example would be how the world appears to someone more optimistic versus someone more pessimistic, in a good mood versus a bad mood, joyful versus fearful, or someone who is open to opportunity versus someone who sees obstacles.

The current position that the person takes is down to social conditioning and their experiences to date, so not their fault at all—we must remove blame, which leads to shame. On realising, there is now a chance to start making that transformation, beginning with the creation of the right habits of thought and action.

The next step is to think about what you will definitely do. The certainty is important because we are often guilty of setting the bar too high (expectations) and delivering low (reality). If you go the other way and set the bar low, maximising your chances of success, then expectations and reality match, keeping motivation going and making it more likely to be repeated. Obviously, repetition is important.

2. Set the bar low

Setting the bar low stacks the probabilities in the favour of succeeding. Remember that getting better requires evidence you are trying to create in what you do. Try to make success the most likely outcome, although you can never be 100%. However, not trying is 100% guaranteed you will get what you don't want!

You can decide now what you will definitely do, and write it down in your journal. For example, I will definitely walk ten minutes each day.

You are confident this is achievable, whereas twenty minutes is more of a 'maybe'. If you are present and aware, you will also notice a feeling of confidence and belief rather than unsure.

When will you practise? Deciding the best time of day and diarising it helps to cement it into your plan.

3. Choose the best time of day to practice

You can stack the new habit onto an existing one. For instance, after breakfast is the time you go for your walk. Or each time you make a cup of coffee, you practise some movements following the principle of one rep is better than none. In other words, by doing one rep of something you have been successful in terms of an approach and attitude, taking one more step in the right direction.

This is a positive action that typically leads to more such actions—you build momentum. This is focusing on the process over the prize and doing the basics well and consistently.

4. Stack your new habit on an established one

Once you have practised, acknowledge your success. A pat on the back to mark what you have done. It feels good.

Feeling good about what you are doing also builds your awareness making it more likely you will think about it at other times during the day. Of course, setting the bar low means that this is the baseline; what you will do each day. If the circumstances allow, you may do more—another set or a few reps. Realising that you have done more than you planned is exceeding your expectations, which is super fuel for positive change.

5. Acknowledge your wins

These are some basic tools for creating a new habit successfully. As humans we often find it difficult to do this and maintain the practice, especially if there is no obvious reward that comes quickly. Keeping your picture of success in mind (read your journal page on this each morning as a reminder) and the reasons why it matters can help. You are trying to live your life according to your values.

Encouragement points

- The quality of your life is greatly determined by your habits.
- We can create new habits of thought and action.
- There are some specific steps you can take to form new habits that are the steps towards your picture of success, including setting the bar low.
- Acknowledge your wins.

Medication and interventions

'Medication and interventions can have a role, but a small one compared to learning and practicing skills to live well and get better.' RS

Medication can be an important part of the treatment process. And whilst I am a proponent of proactively overcoming persistent pain, there can be a role for drugs. People often ask me in our sessions, and I tell them that whilst I know about and understand the different types of drug, this must be managed by your doctor.

Likewise with interventions, there is a place, but only within the bigger picture of you understanding your pain and what you can do to improve your life. The latter is the proactive approach and makes the bulk of what you do to move forward. If medicine and interventions help along the way, this is a plus. But they are not the main thrust of getting better, which is an active process.

This is not a comprehensive look at the different medical options. Instead some observations and thoughts I would like to share with you if and when you are making these kinds of decisions.

What is the purpose of the treatment?

It must be explained to you what the treatment can achieve. What is the point? Or more bluntly, what's in it for me?

What does it do?

Knowing what the treatment may have an impact on how it goes. Many people tell me that they don't know how the intervention works or what it is meant to do. If you can't explain it to someone, you don't understand it. Ultimately, you are having something done to you invasively and putting drugs into your body. Knowing what it can do, what is hoped it will do and the possible side effects are all part of making an informed decision.

Another way to put it is making conscious decisions. This means that you are fully aware of the pluses and minuses, minimising uncertainty and feeling empowered by your choice. This is the same for any decision we make day to day. Knowing that there are always consequences and realising what they could be is at the heart of making the best decisions in most cases.

What are the risks?

All interventions come with a degree of risk. For the clinician administering the treatment it can be routine, but it is certainly not routine for the person on the other end. That must never be taken for granted, and every opportunity to reassure and explain the process is vital.

A conversation about the treatment includes the risk factors. You can weigh these up against possible benefits before making your decision. And it is your decision. If you decide against it, this should be supported and alternatives sought.

In terms of medication, the risks are the side effects. Knowing that there can be side effects is a double-edged sword. Being told that you may experience certain things; could this affect the likelihood of having such experiences? Yes, that is possible. You will have heard of the placebo effect and maybe the nocebo effect.

Medication reviews

If you are taking regular medication as part of your programme, this should be reviewed at regular intervals with your doctor. Preferably the prescriber who knows you and your situation.

Often the doctor initiates a review date, perhaps a few months down the line. It takes time for some of the drugs to take effect and to give you a chance to see how they are helping or not. Some find it useful to keep a note in their journal, although we have to recognise that there is no single factor ever at play. In other words, we look for a simple cause and effect but the reality is that there are many variables in any given moment. Most of these we are unaware of because they are our biology in the dark.

If there is no structure or plan for your medication, I advise you to talk to your doctor to gain clarity. In my opinion, you should know what you are taking, how it works (why you are taking it), and the future plan for reducing and coming off the medication. This is unless the drug is for a particular condition when the plan may be different.

As with interventions and surgery, there is a role for medication. However, it is a small role compared to the skills of living well, skills to deal with challenging moments and those that take you towards your picture(s) of success. Taking medication or having a treatment done to you (i.e. passive) do not teach you how to live or make best decisions at the moment. Getting better and living your best life is a proactive process. A journey you are following with increasing skill, confidence, and independence.

Encouragement points

- Gather as much information as you feel you need in order to make a conscious decision, fully aware of the pluses and minuses.
- Follow the treatment plan as best you can in order to measure the outcomes as accurately as possible.

- Organise a regular medication review with your doctor.
- Ask for a plan if you do not have one.

Building health

'Focus on what you want, for example a healthy life, rather than what you don't want.' RS

One of the bedrocks of improving life and hence overcoming pain is to build health and wellness. The World Health Organisation (WHO) defines health as a state of complete physical, mental, and social well-being and not merely the absence of disease or infirmity (2021). This is a state we can strive to achieve, but always considering that there are circumstances such as living conditions, opportunities for healthy activities, financial constraints and demands, and your social network.

It strikes me as easy to suggest health-giving practices, yet hard for many people to put into practice without the right kind of support. This is one of the reasons why we must consider pain as a social issue, a political issue, and a public health concern. For a person to be relieved, the context of their life must be considered within any treatment and recovery programme.

'Wellness' is defined in the Merriam-Webster dictionary as the quality or state of being in good health, especially as an actively sought goal. Dictionary.com concurs with the quality or state of being healthy in body and mind, especially as the result of deliberate effort. It goes on to add that wellness is an approach to healthcare that emphasises preventing illness and prolonging life, as opposed to emphasising treating diseases. It seems then that the commonality is the active pursuit of a healthy state. In doing so, by focusing on a positive and healthy way of being, you gain the benefits of such habits whilst diminishing the risks of disease and illness.

This is very much in line with the Pain Coach approach to overcoming persistent pain. It is also congruent with the decision and efforts to focus on what you want, rather than what you don't; that is, I want to lead a good life. There can be a tendency for people to tell me initially that their picture of success is to be pain-free or to be relieved somewhat. This is entirely understandable and indeed the programme is designed to ease pain and suffering. However, to have the goal and expectation that you will be pain-free or reduced pain, the focus is on the pain. This is just the same as saying don't think of elephants. What is the first thing you think about?

Essentially, to be successful with anything you need to be clear about what it is you want to achieve. Then you focus on the steps to take right now. By focusing on wanting to be pain-free or relieved of pain, you are actually keeping awareness and attention on the pain, the very thing you don't want. So what can you do instead? Focus on the healthy future you. Why? Because that is what you want to achieve. I know that it sounds simple, and in principle it is.

Yet the human mind works in a different way because the priority is survival. In states of persistent pain, the person is looking out for possible dangers and threats, anticipating that this is a likely explanation for what is happening right now. This is what you want to transform, so that the anticipation is of healthy states, created by repeated practice of the skills of being well.

Health and wellness do not come immediately. They emerge from repeated, daily habits like cleaning your teeth. We brush our teeth several times each day to create the conditions for future oral health. And so as not to put off the person you are speaking to. One day, you don't look at your teeth and think, that's it, I can stop cleaning them now. You keep going, day after day. This is the reality of being healthy; day-to-day practices with no end point. It's a journey.

Creating your healthy daily pillars, you are looking after your future self. Each decision you make is shaping your future. This is why you benefit from knowing the kind of future you want, what matters to you, and why. Then you can make informed decisions, aware of the pluses and minuses of each. If you decide to stay up late, you will not be surprised to feel less energetic the next day, together with being moody and less effective. Some of these decisions do not bear fruit for some time, including those that are important for wellness such as exercise. This can pose a challenge for some people.

When you decide to be more active, you will not feel the benefit the next day. Your body will not appear differently. You may feel good about having made the effort and completed the task, and this is important to note (see Journal). But to see and feel significant change means we have to repeat and repeat, day after day, as we sculpt that future self in what we choose to do now. Similarly, one biscuit today will not make much difference. But if you eat biscuits every day, there will be a consequence in terms of your metabolism and the risk of certain diseases.

You will already have many habits. We all do. These are things we do automatically, without thought. Some argue that the quality of our lives is determined by the quality of our habits. That makes some sense. It also opens an opportunity to change our direction by making different choices.

As humans we seem to find this challenging, but there is good news. You can form new habits (see Habits) to yield desirable results. The first step is to decide that you are going to take action, knowing the reasons why it is important. Now you have the intent and need a plan. I am hoping that you will form that plan and take action off the back of reading and using this book.

More good news is that the habits we can choose from are plentiful and can be thought of as skills. This means you can practise and get better at them. As you do this and the habits take hold, the way that your body systems are working will change. In turn, your experiences will change as the predictions of your state update. You are actively steering yourself towards the healthier version of you by focusing on what you can control.

This is your potential to shape something better. There is no end point to this, as I said. You continue practising for as long as it is important to be well and healthy—is there an end to that? As ever, challenges will arise. But as you build resilience and confidence, you will find that you can increasingly deal with them and there is less impact or suffering.

Being healthy and practising the skills of being well are not an end result. Instead, they are steps along a continuous path.

You will have your own ideas as to what being well is and feels like. This is a good start point from which you can take steps forward. Each practice and choice is another vote for that version of you.

Skills of being well

The work of Richard Davidson, professor of psychology and psychiatry at the University of Wisconsin-Madison, has shown that there are particular skills you can practise and improve, in order to build your wellness. You will be familiar with learning and the need for practice to improve, so it is exciting to think that the same applies to our health.

The four skills Davidson believes can help our well-being are awareness, connection, insight, and purpose. He also calls them qualities. In a recent paper, Davidson and colleagues outlined the framework that the four skills create, describing what is known with regard to brain changes and experiences (Dahl et al., 2020). There are other skills of being well such as exercise, diet, and sleep, but it is both interesting and important to know that the four identified and studied by Davidson can make a difference.

Much of this section will be based on this work, plus other important healthy considerations from science and my practice with people suffering persistent pain.

Before looking at the skills, one of the most important precursors to take on board, as Davidson states, is that 'by nurturing virtuous qualities of mind, we actually can promote positive changes in the brain'. There are actual changes in the nervous system as a result of this kind of training. Now, it is important to say that there are always changes and developments in our body systems, but the direction of that change will depend on our decisions, habits, and the circumstances we find ourselves in.

In other words, there are practices (see Mindfulness) that we can use to cultivate our minds with important healthy results in our brains. But it goes beyond this according to Davidson. He talks about the ability of our behaviour to affect gene expression—that means you as a whole person.

This is the field of epigenetics, which together with neuroplasticity give us explanations for our ability to grow in a particulate direction. This direction obviously depends upon what we practise often. Essentially, neuroplasticity is the object of study for most neuroscience, looking at and understanding what is happening and changing in the nervous system over time.

Davidson and his team have created an app called Healthy Minds, which is a freely available resource that takes you through the practices and teachings based on the skills of being well (awareness, connections, insight, and purpose).

Starting with Davidson's four skills, I then describe others that I have found to be important to people.

Awareness (and attention)

We appear to live in a world of chronic distraction. Our brains have been trained within the context of the digital era and social media to seek novelty over and over (see section Social media). Even a second's opportunity whilst waiting in line must be filled with a quick check of emails or scroll through a feed. The idea of just standing still and being in the moment and our thoughts creates huge discomfort in many people. This is eased with a simple look at one of the many social media platforms.

The opposite of distraction, awareness, means to pay attention and focus. People who can pay attention for longer report being happier than those who are less able (Killington & Gilbert, 2010). You might make a link there between the effects of social media use and your mood, beyond the way that the content you are absorbing is making you feel.

To become more focused and able to be present are interrelated and can be practised. One way is through daily meditation (see Mindfulness). Another way is to construct a way of working that encourages a deeper engagement (see Focus and attention). Cal Newport (2016) digs into the concept of deep work in his book with the same title. He explores ways that you can create and cultivate working practices from where a state of absolute presence and focus emerges. It is in these states, he argues, that you can do your best work, giving many examples of people's successes, backed by research in the field. Whilst this can obviously refer to work as employment, this can also mean the day-to-day tasks you engage with—things you normally do.

To achieve deeper states of focus, you can construct your environment and schedule your time to support your endeavours. For example, you can turn off or put away devices and other things that would distract you, choosing to make them less available. This may be uncomfortable at the start, but remembering what you value and what you are trying to achieve can help. When you pay attention, you soon realise that those feelings pass by, just like all others.

Designing a daily timetable keeps you on track. I encourage you to make a weekly and daily plan (see Planning, prioritising, and periodising) so that you can incorporate all that is necessary and matters into your day. You can tick each activity off as you go, feeling a sense of satisfaction. This also allows you to choose the best times for certain tasks. Some people can focus better in the morning, so this becomes time to do the kind of work that requires your concentration. Chunking your time into manageable slots followed by breaks for recharging, means that you can engage with the job and then pause. This is one of the habits of peak performers.

Deep work delivers results. You are also getting into a great state, which is healthy. The more you are in such states, the more you will be in such states. You are training yourself. Importantly for persistent pain, the more you can be in great states, the less you will be in a protected state. If you do experience pain, because you have been in a flow, you will be better positioned to deal with those moments, as you have more resilience and energy. So, getting into flow by creating the right conditions is an important skill for getting better and shaping a positive future.

Switching off is another important practice that helps you engage in deep work. Often, all waking hours are made available via email, social media, and messaging. It can even go beyond this as many people have their phones by their bed. Just in case. Undoubtedly there have been times when someone has called in the night because of an emergency. But how often does this actually happen versus the number of times you check your email or another well-known social media app? Some questions on this:

- Do you check you phone as soon as you get up?
- Do you check your phone last thing before bed?
- Do you check your phone if you wake up in the night?
- Do you check your phone if you are waiting for something, to fill the time?
- Why?

Each time you check, it evokes some kind of feeling that is underpinned by a change in body chemistry. Your brain predicts that by checking your phone, you will feel better, easing the discomfort that has arisen from seemingly doing nothing, or that there may be some kind of reward: a like. With this quick fix, it becomes an immediate reward. Feeling good, you do it again and again.

But, there can also be the stress response triggered by checking social media. If you have not received any likes, the content you consume is toxic or you receive a negative message, your biology changes in readiness to fight, run away, or freeze (see Managing stress). How many times does this happen to you? Whatever we train and practise, we get better at. The habits you have to date are delivering your current experiences. If they are not the ones you want, you can create new habits for a healthier version of you (see Habits).

To switch off then, becomes an important way to change state and recharge. Put another way, if you were asked: 'There is something simple you can do to reduce stress in your life and build wellness, are you interested?', how would you respond?

There are many ways to switch off, and you will already know some, or perhaps you have already incorporated this practice into your life. Here are some suggestions:

- When you get up, use a morning routine (see section) of breathing and movement before you check your phone.
- Set a time for your first and last phone check.
- Have a day off social media each week.
- Choose certain hours each day when you do not check email or social media.

As you can see, they are simple. The key is to have the intent and to know why it matters to you. Then create your habit so it is achievable and acknowledge your wins along the way.

Strengthening your self-awareness helps you to better regulate your emotions. Dahl et al. (2020) describe lower stress levels, less reactivity to pain, more positivity, and well-being as a result of practising mindfulness as a way to improve attention and self-awareness.

There is only one moment, and it is this one. To be present means that you are here in the now rather than somewhere else and distracted. Whether you are doing a piece of work or listening to a loved one, if you are present you are able to notice what is actually happening and respond skilfully. To be absent, on the other hand, means you are missing the opportunities. We have all had the experience of talking to someone who is distracted versus someone who is deeply listening. Which feels better?

Connections

It is accepted that the quality of our connections plays a significant role in our quality of life and our wellness. Consider how it feels when you are with someone who inspires or encourages you. What is the knock-on effect? When you feel good, how are you with others?

Suffering persistent pain can certainly create difficulties in relationships. Changes in the way you feel, your mood, and how you communicate with others can all add strain. I would say, coming through the compassionate focused lens, that this is not your fault. You are not doing this on purpose. Instead, these are the consequences of being in prolonged pain. Also, by finding it hard to participate in the same way means that the dynamics of relationships can shift. When you are socialising less, stop playing sports or work, there are fewer interactions, resulting in less opportunity to nourish the bonds. This takes a new kind of effort and in a different way.

I have dedicated a section to reconnection as this is at the heart of some of the most important practices. Similar to getting into the best states by creating the right conditions as outlined above, reconnecting with people will also cultivate those states. We are designed to connect and co-operate, so tapping into this natural way of being is a powerful antidote to suffering. A loved one showing caring with touch, a word, or a simple presence can be soothing, especially the latter (see Family and friends).

Loved ones and close friends can play an important role in your recovery. But so can other people you know, if you are open to their caring concern or practical support. For example, an understanding boss, a helpful neighbour, or a compassionate therapist. Beyond this are people you don't actually know but you believe can contribute to your success. This could be someone you listen to, watch, or read their words. Nowadays it is easy to immerse yourself in the works of many people: thinkers, spiritual leaders, coaches.

On a lighter note, you can also connect with people who make you laugh; comedians. A quick look online and you will find excerpts of stage shows or TV programmes featuring someone you enjoy listening to and hopefully bringing on a giggle (it may even hurt!). Notice this change of state and how quickly it emerges in you. A dose of this each day can be a wonderful antidote. In fact, so much so in the case of Norman Cousins, he recovered from a severe connective tissue disease that he was told he would have little chance of overcoming. Cousins documented his experience in the book: Anatomy of an illness as perceived by the patient (1979).

Essentially, after the medical treatment failed to help, Cousins set about his own programme that consisted of high doses of vitamin C and watching funny TV programmes and films. He said, 'I made the joyous discovery that ten minutes of genuine belly laughter had an anaesthetic effect and would give me at least two hours of pain-free sleep.' Now, this did cause some controversy. The medical community was not happy that a journalist declared his recovery was due to something else. He was criticised for publishing his story, some claiming that Cousins' improvement was natural, regardless of what he did.

Perhaps there is some truth in this, as there is always a time factor. However, Cousins certainly created conditions that can be argued are ideal for the body to heal. Reducing stress and experiencing great states (mirth, joy, pleasure) would have a positive effect on the inflammatory processes that were contributing to his sensitised state.

So, just as you can take your pills, you can take your 'laughter medication'. One is more natural, sustainable, and safer. There is also no upper limit to how much you can laugh or smile. It is infectious, in a great way.

Music is another way to connect. You may have favourite artists you enjoy listening to or sharing the experience with others. Throughout the day, you may have moments when you put on a particular song or album. If you can move and dance along (in your own way), even better! But don't worry if you can't. Perhaps you can go to a live gig or watch a musical show on the TV with friends and family. This can be a positive experience for everyone, creating a good story to build upon.

There are many ways to connect with loved ones and people we admire. The more we can do this each day, the more we practise being in better states as we seek to move forward. Perhaps you can think of ways you can spend time with people so that everyone benefits from each other's company. It may not be exactly as you wish, but there is always a starting point. For example, using online tools to talk to and see people may not be the perfect option, but it makes something possible. This is very much in line with the principle of thinking about what you can do in line with your picture of success, and stepping on from there (i.e. focus on what you can do rather than what you can't).

Following a positive experience with others, you can note down in your journal what went well, the principles that you followed, and how it felt. Logging your successes allows you to study them and build onwards. This can help to shape your outlook, the way in which you see your future, an important motivator.

Insight

How well do you know yourself? How self-aware are you at any given moment? It seems that the more insight we have into our sense of self and the types of things we tell ourselves make a difference.

This is one of the effects of consistent meditation practice. You come to know your own (embodied) mind and your tendencies, putting you in a position to make better decisions. We can argue that the quality of your decisions affects the quality of your life.

Of course, you don't need to necessarily meditate to gain this insight. Stopping and reflecting on what you have thought and done or journaling can also build your awareness of how you do things. Ultimately, you create opportunities to be better at what you are doing each day. In a coaching sense, this is the definition of success: being better today than yesterday, and repeating this every day. Dr Stephen Fleming, head of the Metacognition Lab at University College London gives a superb account of the research on self-awareness in his recent book, Know Thyself.

Purpose

This is your reason to get up in the morning. Simon Sinek calls it your 'why?', and Seth Godin your 'caring', which is a play on calling. Essentially it is what you care about and hence act upon. There can be more than one, of course. For instance, a parent, a partner, a friend, a worker, a contributor. You might like to spend a moment thinking about what you really care about in your life.

Purpose has long been known to be an important part of a healthy life. The opposite is also true. One of the disconnects that people often describe to me when they are telling me about their life is a loss of purpose. They are not doing the things that they used to, because of the pain and fear of the pain. This detachment is felt in many ways, including loneliness when a purpose revolves around being with other people. Now the person finds themself apart from others and what they want to be able to do. This highlights the fact that many of these parts of life are interrelated.

How can you reconnect with your purpose? The way this looks may well have changed. Examples include your purpose as a parent, a partner, a friend, how you contribute to a project, or something else. Notice how these are all things that you care about. Reconnecting with them bit by bit is part of getting better.

It is understandable to think about what has been lost and the things that you cannot do. Of course, this will feel bad. The practice and skill of switching your focus to what you can do and how you can move forward takes some effort but is possible. That is my encouragement to you.

Using the practice and strategies in this book you can reconnect with what matters and work towards your pictures of success, and with a new sense of purpose. Naturally, shaping a positive future often becomes one of the main purposes.

Compassion, gratitude, kindness to others

Your outlook, or how you think that things will turn out for you, will affect the types of things that you do. Hope is tied closely with this, emerging from your belief in your own ability to get better, improve your life, and ease your pain. The weighting as to which is more important to you will determine your actions. This is why understanding your pain is a key first step (see What is pain?—always good to reread and review this section to deepen your knowledge). Knowing that you are safe to be active whilst acknowledging that there are better ways to do this (e.g. pace, take breaks, gradually build your window of tolerance) will be very different from fearing pain means harm or injury.

The way that the science and philosophy of pain are progressing gives great hope. This must be transmitted to society and individuals to harness the knowledge in practical ways. Whilst you may be suffering right now, knowing that this will pass and that you can feel better is powerful. The opposite feeling, hopelessness, whilst reasonable under the circumstances of fear and in the face of repeated failures to ease symptoms, usually results in modest ongoing efforts.

This is one of the reasons why I often see people perk up when we talk about their pain, what is actually happening, and what they can do to actively move forward. Knowing there is a way gives hope because your outlook changes.

Other skills of being well

There are many to choose from and will largely depend on what you want to achieve—your picture(s) of success. Having said that, there are some that we all need to be well: a good sleep habit, diet, and exercise (whatever form best works for you; could also be called activity that involves some kind of movement).

Throughout the sections, you will come across a range of skills that you can practise in order to build your wellness as part of the journey onwards. The day-to-day habits we have are creating the conditions for a particular future. What is that future? What does it look like for you? What habits and skills must you use in order for that particular future to manifest?

Building health

These and the other practices described in the book are the bricks. With the bricks, you build your own house on strong foundations of understanding. This in itself requires a strategy and know-how. I bring this together in the final section with the same title.

Fundamentally, health is built by consistent, day-to-day practices in the same way that they are important to overcome pain. This means creating habits (see Habits).

One of the difficulties we have as humans is acting now for an unseen benefit. We like quick rewards. However, the important things in life don't work this way. They take time and persistence, with no end point in sight. Think relationships, work satisfaction, and health. A simple example I often use is cleaning your teeth. Whilst you may like the minty taste, the reason you do it twice a day is for future oral health. You are managing your future in what you do now.

Encouragement points

- Building health is an active, daily process featuring certain habits that create the conditions for a future you.
- There are skills of being well, meaning that we can all practise certain things to get results.

- The skills of being well are part of a way of overcoming pain, together with specific practices, exercises, tools, and strategies.
- As with any skill, when you practise, you get better at it.
- This is one way of feeling more in control—you are focusing on what you can control and on process over prize.

Managing stress

'Stress is less about what is happening and more about how you relate to it. This you can update and ease your own suffering.' RS

The way you manage stress will govern how the ups and downs are for you. Some people seem able to roll with most things that happen to them, whilst others have great difficulty. It is very individual and largely down to how you have been conditioned to see the world. You are familiar with the compassionate approach now, to understand that it is not the person's fault the way they respond, but that they can gain insights and learn better ways.

Persistent pain itself can be stressful. Whilst there will be an individual way of experiencing this, I think we can all agree that the impact and the actual nature of what it is like to be suffering pain will cause stress. Even with other aspects of life being manageable or good, the pain will typically be stressful. Unfortunately for many people suffering persistent pain, life is stressful in many other ways, then amplified by the pain and the effects of it ongoing.

The kinds of problems people encounter include limited or loss of work with a knock-on financial impact, relationship difficulties, loss of identity, a dwindling social life, and an inability to play sports or exercise to name but a few. You suffer the effects of loss and less, often fearing losing out further. Essentially, at the heart of this is a disconnection from what matters in your life, which is why reconnecting is such a vital part of shaping a positive future (see Reconnection).

There are many causes of stress depending on the person. You probably know the kinds of things that bring on the familiar feelings. Like all feelings, they are our perceptions and in a predictive sense, the best explanation for what is happening right now in our lived world, based on previous experiences.

When you feel a certain way, being in a given state, it becomes what it is because of the label we give to the feeling. Before that, it is just a feeling. Seeing this is an important step in learning to manage stress better. You are not choosing to respond in the way you do, it has been learned. And now you want to learn another way.

It is so that in our society, permissive ways of dealing with stress include alcohol, cigarettes, and shopping. Certainly, people should not be judged for using such methods to meet their needs. If someone else were in their shoes, they would most likely be doing the same. Other choices are not apparent or available. This is why just giving up smoking is very difficult without a new habit to replace the old and a strong purpose.

The problem with these ways of dealing with stress is that they are short-lived. In other words, there is no transformation of suffering because they do not deal with the causes of stress. So each time the feeling arises, the quick fix is reached for, quelling the difficulties somewhat and just for now. Then it starts again, building over time. Similar to ongoing pain, there is a stickiness to stress.

To get a sense of this, you may like to think about something that always seems to cause you stress. Has it been this way for a long time? Do you tend to get stressed over the same things now that you have done for years? Would you like to transform this so that you suffer less?

Stress and health

Much has been written on the effects of stress on our health. I will not be providing a comprehensive review here. If you want to understand this in more detail, I encourage you to read the work of Robert Sapolsky, who wrote 'Why Zebras Don't Get Ulcers'. This is a superb account of stress by arguably the world's leading authority.

In short, stress is useful in short bursts. It is a response that enables us to maximise our chances of survival. You have probably heard of flight or fight—run away from danger or fight it. The biological response is in anticipation of the threat, mobilising body systems in preparation, felt as tension in the body, an alertness, and perhaps anxiety amongst other things. In addition to flight or fight, there is also a freeze reaction. Think rabbit in headlights, or when someone is immobilised by fear. These three are adaptive and useful, primarily driven by the SNS. This is one of the branches of the ANS, the other being the parasympathetic.

The problems occur when the stress response is repeatedly activated, essentially flooding our body systems with chemicals such as cortisol. The knock-on effects over time impact on all body systems, which is why you can see wide-ranging symptoms, including aches and pains. When someone comes to see me with a persistent pain problem, it is common that in the conversation they reveal other issues. For instance, headaches, migraines, irritable bowel syndrome

(IBS), pelvic pain, vulvodynia (females), poor concentration, disturbed sleep, low mood, more emotional, fatigue, and general malaise.

I have often described life-itis, with the 'itis' referring to inflammation. Chronic stress switches us into being chronically inflamed, which is the likely biological contribution to this lived experience. Inflammation is the start of healing, and in preparation for the threat to our body integrity, this is set to 'on' and ready just in case. The way we live in the modern world seems to be contributing to this, hence life-itis. Work demands, the pressures to be and look a certain way, social media, less sleep, diet, and the pace of life all contribute. There is often not enough downtime, reflection, insight into how things really are, switching off, self-care, or self-compassion.

The impact of chronic stress is not overnight. It builds slowly over time. A meal of junk food once will have little effect, but if it becomes regular will put strain on the body's systems. Similarly, not moving regularly will not cause immediate problems aside from short-term discomfort. Continue for months and years, your body health takes a hit and moving becomes increasingly challenging.

At any time we can stop and review our habits and make a choice. Each is a vote for who we will become if we continue. Clarifying your picture of success gives you the direction you want to go, and then you can decide which habits are working for you and which are not. This together with learning and practising better ways to deal with stress can direct you towards a healthier future.

The nature of threat

Although the perception of threat is a personal interpretation of what is happening or what could happen, we would all agree that certain situations as causing stress. For example, the loss of a loved one, coping with a serious disease, an abusive relationship, or substandard living conditions.

Then there are future threats that you find yourself responding to now in thought and feeling, wherever you are. This is anxiety—a feeling about an imagined future. Sat on a beach, looking out to sea from a beautiful island, it is quite possible to feel terrible inside because of something you are thinking about, which is not actually happening. This causes a stress response in just the same way, with resources mobilised to deal with the possible threat as if it is actually going to happen. But you are on a beach. In case you are thinking, 'But I am not on a beach', it is the same wherever you find yourself thinking.

The stories we tell ourselves are so convincing that we embody it as if it is happening, completely forgetting where we actually are and what we are actually doing. It is so compelling and powerful that in some cases it could result in a panic attack, which is an extremely unpleasant and often frightening experience.

A threat, real or imagined, will evoke strong biological responses that shape our experiences day to day. Like anything that happens over and over, it becomes a habit, or way of seeing the world. Anxiety and depression are both rife in the modern world, causing much suffering. The number of people who endure these conditions is growing, especially in the younger age groups. It is essential that we get to grips with this problem and help people in practical ways.

Stress and pain

People often make the look between stress and pain themselves when they think about when they feel worse. It is perfectly possible and understandable to have more pain when you are stressed. Both pain and stress are about perceived or predicted threats to your body integrity.

However, it is not always as clear cut as this, and we should not make assumptions. In some cases people feel less or no pain when they are stressed. It really depends on context and the meaning of the situation. It can be that the person is so focused on dealing with the threat, that pain is simply not happening. Also, it is not that pain is somehow lurking in the shadows. You are either in pain or not—it is binary. You are in one state or another. There are plenty of day-to-day examples of this, from battlefield stories to the sports field.

Pain being a perception, experienced by the person in their world, is shaped by many factors including your beliefs, mood, where your attention is placed, expectations, and past experiences, as you now know. So if escaping from the war zone is necessary, there is no point in feeling pain that would only slow you down or risk being caught. This is borne out in the records from battlefield hospitals when soldiers would arrive, reporting little to no pain. You may also have heard stories of sports people finishing a game, only to discover that they have an injury.

I once turned my ankle during an ultramarathon, some 40k into the run. At around 70k I started to feel some discomfort, but put it down to the time on my feet. I finished the race, which was 100k, and crashed out at the accommodation where I was staying. The next morning I woke up feeling very stiff and sore as to be expected. As I walked to the bathroom, I realised that I was limping. Looking down I noticed a blackened and swollen ankle. I hadn't realised until now!

Ways to manage stress

Arguably, skills to manage stress are some of the most important we can learn. Throughout this book, there are tips and tools that you can use, especially in the Challenging moments section. Anything that you do to self-soothe, calm down, and gain insight into what is really happening and then make your next best choice is managing stress.

There will always be ups and downs. Especially when dealing with a persistent pain problem that can affect most if not all areas of life. It seems that the more flexible we can be with our thinking and emotions, be able to see the bigger picture, to distance ourselves from our narrative, and cultivate equanimity, the better the ride we have. Indeed, knowing that you have the skills to deal with stress gives you confidence and a belief in your own ability to cope.

You can be both proactive and reactive to stress. The more you use practices to create calm and clarity, to be present and self-aware, the quicker you will realise when things are building. Recognising and knowing the triggers helps you to intervene before the emotions take hold. Daily meditation and mindful practice can help develop this ability as well as be more skilful ways of responding rather than reacting automatically.

On noticing that you are starting to feel stressed or having the foresight that a particular situation could be stressful, you can use your practices. As you read through the sections, you can make a note of the tools that you will use and how well they work for you.

Encouragement points

- Stress is normal and in the short term is an adaptive response to help you deal with a threatening situation.
- If stress persists, it has an impact on our health over time.
- We can learn skills and practices to better manage stress.
- Managing stress is an important part of building wellness, which in turn is one of the ways you can overcome pain and shape a positive future.

- There are many tools and practices throughout this book. If you like, you can note down the ones you are going to practise and review them moving forward.

Gratitude

'Gratitude is a simple and low-tech practice that is proving to have powerful effects on wellbeing.' RS

When you read or listen to people who have achieved great success, they will talk about their gratitude for certain aspects of their life. Perhaps it is for the people they have known, their parents, the fact that they have a life to live, or something more simple such as the breath. The Pain Coaching approach draws upon the habits of successful people and peak performers, believing that we are all able to use such habits in our day-to-day life to get results. You can learn from others' success and your own.

Gratitude has been studied as a practice because it seems to be something important for our health. Research has been demonstrating such benefits and confirming it as a useful tool. One of the best-known researchers is Robert Emmon who talks of two parts to the practice (2010). Firstly, you affirm some good things exist in the world, despite other more challenging situations and suffering. Secondly, you recognise that the sources of gratitude are coming from the world or other people (2010).

Appreciating other people is a skill of being well that contributes to how you can connect with others, fostering relationships that support your health. You will see this in the Building Health section. Depending on how you have been socially conditioned to look at life, you may see possibilities or problems, or, opportunities or obstacles. It is useful to realise which way you are going. It may vary in different situations of course, and who you are with can have a bearing. Once you have this insight, you can start practising appreciation to shape a different way of seeing the world. It takes time and repetition, but considering the fact that science tells us you see the world you expect to see, it seems to be worth the practice. How far you move along the line will vary, but anything you practise well, you will become better at doing.

We can also look out for things to appreciate in the world. Perhaps the warmth of the sun, the taste of coffee, the sound of music, or something else that gives you energy. Making a list can be helpful, and then setting your intention to look out for them and take a moment to enjoy the perception. Pausing to notice is also a chance to be present, another skill of being well. We must go beyond it just being a thought or a tick-box exercise. So when you put your attention on the subject of appreciation and gratitude, notice how you feel. This makes it whole and a change of state.

Emmons and other researchers have found that people who have cultivated gratitude, including keeping a gratitude journal for just three weeks, demonstrated a host of positive effects (2010). They included better sleep, more positive emotions, feeling greater pleasure and joy, felt more optimistic, were compassionate and generous, and less lonely. Not a bad selection!

It is simple enough in principle, but in practice it is as hard as creating any new habit. We can try to make it part of how we go about our life—a way of being. But sometimes you may forget. That's ok, you are trying to do your best. Notice how it makes you feel so that it goes beyond just a thought.

You will have your own experience, and I hope it is a good one. Interestingly, recent research suggests that the good feelings associated with gratitude could stem from our natural opioids (Henning et al., 2017). In this state, there are certain brain patterns that have been studied (Karns et al., 2017; Fox et al., 2015), although as you know, we are more than a brain. The feelings are embodied and relate to the situation you are in and prior experiences.

Practices

1. At the end of each day, write down three things you are grateful for, think about them, and notice how you feel.
2. As you go about your day, look out for something to be grateful for or appreciate.
3. Before you meet or see someone, think about something you appreciate about them. Then notice how you feel when you are together and how the interaction goes.

Encouragement points

- Practicing gratitude can have a positive effect on your health.
- It is important to focus on the subject of appreciation and to feel it, to make it a whole experience that is marked.
- You can practise on the go, looking out for things you are grateful for, or you can write down 2–3 things you appreciate at the end of the day.

Pauses

'Pauses through the day bring calm and clarity, applying a natural brake to see what is actually happening and to recharge.' RS

You may have heard the phrase 'we are human beings, not human doings'. Somewhere along the line, being busy and non-stop became valued. Fast-paced living, working long hours, and being constantly occupied have all become synonymous with being successful. Of course, it very much depends on your definition of a successful life. And your definition depends in turn on how you have been conditioned to think about living. The people you model and who influence you play a huge role in this together with the society and culture you live within.

In other words, your way of being has been shaped by many external factors and experiences to date. The question now is whether your way actually works for you. Does it deliver the results and kind of life you want to live? Also, what is the cost to you and people close to you?

Together with busyness can be rushing. Many people seem to be in a rush to get where they are going, both literally and metaphorically. Some just do not want to be where they are, believing that to be somewhere else will be better when they eventually get there—the grass is greener. Whether it be walking or driving, commonly people are speeding along, often not present but lost in thought. Getting caught up in a whirlwind of tasks, little time to do them and being on autopilot is a route of persistent stress and often unhappiness compared to being able to spend more time paying attention and being present.

Someone might work very long hours, be dedicated to their company, bring work home in the evenings and at weekends, and successfully deliver projects. However, the cost could be a lack of time with the family and friends, minimal time to be active, poor diet, and disrupted sleep. Whilst work may continue to go well, other areas of life gradually deteriorate. Ultimately, the prized work will be affected because without health and wellness, sustained performance becomes impossible.

A parent may try to ensure that everyone else in the family's needs are met on a daily basis. They keep themselves at the bottom of the pile. Others coming first is a common message drilled into people from an early age. Of course, caring for other people is a wonderful thing to do, but can only be sustained if you look after yourself. This is a challenge for many people—self-caring and self-compassion. They are important for your well-being.

Many people have told me that their parents, often their mothers, used to care for everyone, but not themselves so much. They were shown this way together with messages about self-caring being selfish. But it is not selfish. It is important for the person and those close by who are influenced. A shift in thinking and a nurturing of compassionate practices day to day is vitally needed in our modern world (see Compassion).

Being on the go without breaks and time to rest and recharge can result in prolonged or chronic stress. As scientist and stress expert, Professor Robert Sapolsky said: 'We live well enough to have the luxury to get ourselves sick with purely social, psychological stress' (A Primate's Memoir). He seems to like the word luxury. Sapolsky also described the deadliest diseases as those that are characterised by gradual damage accumulating over time; 'the luxury of slowly falling apart', he said.

We have looked at stress previously. Most people realise stress is a personal response. Whether a situation is stressful or not depends on the meaning that you give to it. You will have some automatic reactions that have been learned. On realising these, you can learn new responses that are more skilful as we have discussed. The way you relate to a situation matters in terms of what it is like for you.

One simple way to counter the issue of always being a human 'doing' is to bring pauses into the day. Undoubtedly, some people have many demands upon them. This can be one of the reasons for not self-caring of course. That might be you, wondering how you are going to be able to do all the things you need to. And then bringing pauses into the day! There is just no time. Perhaps another way to put it is thinking of the cost of not slowing down at times. What will be the cost to you? In a month? A year? Five years; how will you be in five years if you do not look after yourself more skilfully and consistently? What does that look like and how does it feel now as you imagine it?

Typically in the clinic, we would have a discussion about this, as I come to understand your world. Then we look for opportunities to introduce healthy practices throughout the day. You have already seen how it works better to use skills and tools at different times of the day rather than all in one go. You wouldn't eat all your meals when you get up and then not bother for the rest of the day. Same with exercises and practices to overcome pain by living a better and better life.

What are pauses?

Pauses are short breaks when you take a moment to be present and aware of what is happening to you. They are an opportunity to check in to see how you are and to meet your needs. Doing this more often than not means you are looking after yourself and your health, even if you simply get yourself a drink when you are thirsty versus ignoring the need. Or not being aware in the first place through being on autopilot.

Stopping and slowing down gives you another set of gears. This allows you greater flexibility to deal with ups and downs, much like cycling a bike over hilly terrain. It is a more comfortable and sustainable ride with more than one or two gears.

Having a brief break, although sometimes longer (e.g. lunch break, mid-morning breaks), not only affords relief, it also gives you the opportunity to practise a healthy habit. Each time you do this, you are shaping a healthier future. Of course, this needs consistency over days, weeks, and months. But every practice is a step in your desired direction.

Longer pauses are also important. We can draw on the habits of peak performers and people like Tom Rath who has studied what matters for health. Rath has not only been dealing with his own serious health challenges for many years but has also been a major contributor to other people's self-care practices. An advocate for strengths coaching, he recognised the importance of taking responsibility for and managing one's own health.

Rath faced his own cancer. In *Eat, Move, Sleep* he says:

> *'I first started doing this research to save my own life, literally. While I have been reluctant to discuss this before, I have been battling cancer for more than twenty years now.'*

One of Rath's personal goals was to live longer than was expected. To do this he needed to examine his way of living and discover healthy practices that would increase his chances. This was not about survival, however, through his work he wanted to thrive and to contribute. A later book, Life's Great Question (2020) looks at how you can live a meaningful life based upon the words of Dr. Martin Luther King, Jr: 'Life's most persistent and urgent question is: What are you doing for others?' This ties neatly with the importance of reconnecting with your purpose (See Reconnection) as health giving.

Rath and many others have highlighted the importance of movement for health (see Movement). Essentially, we need movement to punctuate our day to achieve goals and to nourish our body and body systems. Pauses enable us to bring regular and consistent changes of position or particular movements into our day. The longer pauses are when we might also be recharging (eating, a brief nap, reading) or taking extended exercise (e.g. a walk, a class, gym, online session). This kind of pattern is often used by peak performers. These are people who consistently produce high-quality work.

The great news is that we can all use the habits of peak performers. The way you organise your day is an important part of following through because it gives you a structure to follow. For instance, some performers will work in chunks of 45–90 minutes before pausing and having a break of 10-15 minutes. This is repeated throughout the day, with the time chunks filled with different tasks and activities (see Planning).

The pauses between the time chunks are as important as the work or the practice. This is when you give yourself the opportunity to adapt and recharge, ready for the next job.

How to remember?

When you have planned your day, it becomes more likely that you will take pauses as planned. Diarising your schedule can increase this likelihood until it becomes a habit—the planning and the execution.

Some people find it useful to have a reminder or to set notifications. One that I often recommend is the Mindful Bell from the Plum Village app. Plum Village is a monastic community in France founded by Thich Nhat Hanh. Throughout the day, the bell is rung and on hearing the sound, everybody stops what they are doing. Using a breathing awareness practice, each member of the community becomes present. Then they continue with their activities. Plum Village has created an app that contains teachings, practices, and much more, including the bell that you can set to ring throughout your day. You can find more here: https://plumvillage.app/

Your plan

Each person will have their own timings according to their current capability and reality. Different activities will have different timelines, so your chunks will be shorter and longer accordingly.

As you progress, your timings will change, but the pauses and breaks remain in place after each. This is a dynamic process that needs regular reviewing and updating.

Examples

1. A popular practice to use for short pauses is breathing awareness. For 2–3 breaths, you sit upright and relaxed, or as comfortably as you can, and follow your breath in and out. This may then lead to another practice or you return to your prior activity.

2. Changing your posture. If you have been sitting, one of the reasons for discomfort is the pressure on the backs of your thighs and buttocks. Blood flow slows in the tissues, the oxygen levels drop, and acid levels rise. This can become uncomfortable or painful. Moving by shifting your posture or standing up allows restoration of blood flow and often relief. The key as ever is to try and do this before you have to and to be consistent.

3. Choose a movement or two or three, depending on the situation. But one is always better than none! This could be a stretch, a walk, a yoga pose, or another movement that you know and like. Some people if they are able, enjoy jumping up and down on the spot. This often feels energising when you stop after 10–20 seconds to feel your body. Building a library of different movements gives you a range of options to consider throughout the day. Variety is good, as are those movements that replicate things we do in our lives. Dancing is also popular, which accompanied by singing can give a real lift.

4. A drink or a snack.

5. Mindful practice (see Mindfulness).

6. Something that brings you joy or pleasure. There is a huge importance of this practice to shift your perspective and make progress. It has its own section (see Joyful activities).

Encouragement points

- Pauses are an important part of your daily programme.
- They provide an opportunity to practice a skill of being well.
- This is a moment to check in and meet your needs.
- Slowing down and recharging is essential for sustained health.

Living life

'Undoubtedly, from listening to people who have overcome their pain, living life is the best pain killer. By focusing on valued activities and dealing skilfully with whatever comes up.' RS

One of the main principles of Pain Coaching is to live life. This is sometimes a challenging message to read or hear, so I will explain it in more detail so you can understand. Of course, you want to live your life, and you are trying your best.

Traditionally, when someone is suffering pain, the so-called source of that pain is sought in terms of a structure, a pathology or something else that can be seen on a test. What and whether anything is found depends upon the test itself to an extent, and the person or system that analyses the results. As you probably know, in many cases there is nothing significant found and certainly nothing that explains the pain and suffering.

When you understand pain, you know that tests never show pain (you cannot see it) and that if something is seen on a test, the relationship to pain varies enormously. Multiple studies have shown this variability yet society continues to predominantly use a model that searches for objective evidence as the evidence. If nothing is found, there are mixed messages given to people. For example, it is psychosomatic, or psychological.

Sometimes there are signs of inflammation or an injury ('damage') and this is used to explain the pain. This makes sense in our world as it is the model we have grown up with over many years. But this does not actually explain the experience of pain. You simply cannot reduce pain to anything less than the person—it is the person who feels pain, not the body part (I say this over and over!).

This is not to ignore findings, but instead to take them as part of the bigger picture to be able to give meaning to your experience of pain. We must incorporate your lived experiences and any scientific knowledge. The biomedical model does not explain pain as it is far too simple. Predictive processing provides explanations for both the subjective and objective findings, as well as a way forward, which is why I come through this lens for now.

As a consequence of reducing pain to a body part or system, there is an implication and assumption that an intervention can be directed to that region. Again, this makes sense because of our existing beliefs about pain and the way the body works. We have been led to think that our bodies are like a computer that can be fixed when it goes wrong. A part goes awry and we can remove it or replace it, just like a machine. Except we are not like that at all! There is no fixing in my opinion, only creating the conditions to build health and wellness. To think fixing is to go down the wrong path with the wrong expectations in many cases.

Some readers may be thinking that people do get fixed surely? What about a hip replacement? Or surgery that literally fixes a broken bone into place. I would still say that these very skilled procedures are about creating the conditions for a more integral body, which when predicted as such will be less likely to be painful. Healing process is an incredibly powerful process in the body that is mainly run by the immune system, although other systems are involved—no system works in isolation. In fact, you are better to think about a nervous-immune-endocrine ensemble working for you to restore your biology to healthy parameters.

Following on down the traditional (biomedical) path, it is assumed that the pain can be treated by addressing the 'bit' that is seen to be faulty. Your whole experience is simply put down to a small part of you going wrong, in this way of thinking. I am hoping you can see the issue with this limited view. There will be people who do feel that their experience of pain was successfully treated this way. I have seen and heard them. But then I ask why they have come to see me, as they are still suffering.

Recovery is a matter of treating the pain by doing something to the body (I would say to the person). Now, this may be an important part of getting better, but it is certainly not the only way. The temptation for many who take this route is to believe that once their pain is better or resolved, then they can start living. This is the view that I would challenge as a fundamental part of the Pain Coaching approach. The main issue is that to wait for something to happen before you start living life, is that you could be waiting an awfully long time, especially if you are relying on treatment 'being done to you' for your pain.

So what can you do instead?

Together, we can turn this model on its head and say, let's get back to living by living, not waiting for something to happen. With this approach, there is intent, empowerment, and a positive way forward. Of course, each person is free to choose their way, and this is one suggestion.

I frequently say to people: when the focus is on treating the pain, the outcomes are poor. But when the focus is on the life you want to live and the steps to take to get there, the outcomes are much better. You are choosing to move your life forward using new knowledge, skills, practices, and know-how, step by step. People are often surprised when I tell them the things they can do to get better and improve their pain are the things that they normally love to do. We just need to look at the best ways of doing them now, considering the circumstances, and build on a baseline that has been established.

I hope that this makes sense to you.

The Pain Coaching approach is to clarify your picture(s) of success and then create a practical series of daily steps, or habits, that take you that way.

How does it work?

You may be wondering how this way helps with your pain. It may help to understand (along with your new knowledge from the 'What is pain?' section) that when you are feeling pain, you are in a particular state biologically and in terms of having an experience. When you are in a different state, there is a different feel. For example, if you are with a loved one laughing, or fully immersed in a film. When you are not in pain, that is also a particular state.

Instead of focusing on the pain and trying to relieve it directly, which is also an approach and can be part of your way of course, you can seek to get into better states by the things you choose to engage with. These things are the ones that matter to you. They can tie in with your values, which you have thought about and listed now. For example, one of your values could be living a healthy life. In light of this, you make many decisions based on your health and create the conditions for the future healthy version of you. What you choose to eat, being active in your own way, connecting with people in encouraging relationships and meditating could form part of your way of manifesting health. These are things that are important to you, because your health is important to you.

Taking this forward, you build your day according to these principles. You are focusing on how you want to be, healthy and well, rather than upon pain. Now, persistent pain can simply arise like all other appearances in consciousness (what you see, feel, smell, etc.), seemingly unbidden. There is nothing you have to do per se to feel pain. It just happens under certain conditions and when you are in certain states. Therefore, filling your day with chosen activities and those that need to be undertaken (perhaps work, chores, caring for children), which are meaningful and purposeful, means you will be in other and hopefully better states.

Stringing these together through the day means you are intentionally living, albeit in particular ways that are planned and periodised for now. This highlights the importance of organising your time well, with the rest and recharge breaks. Doing the basics like this consistently well means that you will be able to organically increase the time you are active. In other sections you will develop your knowledge of how and when to progress, remembering the principle of impermanence and that you always have the potential to improve your life.

Ways to live your life

This is very individual, but I will share some ideas that I commonly discuss with the people I work with. Naturally you begin by talking about the types of things that you like and love to do, thinking about how they make you feel. This can be hard, of course, because the mind can drift to the fact that you may not be doing those things. But then you can turn our attention to how you can re-engage (see Reconnection).

You are free to design your life within the parameters of what you are able to do within a particular environment. When thinking about your future life, which is anything beyond now and never actually reached, you can draw out your ideal. This may or may not be how it turns out, but you are putting your energy into it and giving it your best shot. You cannot ask more of yourself. Being clear, then, is important for direction and acts as a reference point when you drift off course.

Having designed your future life (picture of success), you can then decide upon the daily practices and habits that you need. Some of these you will already be doing, and you can build on them.

1. Choosing things that matter

Assuming that you have planned and periodised your day to meet your needs and considering your circumstances right now (reality), you can now decide what will fill the chunks of time. If it is a working day, you will have time doing your job divided up and punctuated with movement, breathing, or another practice that is nourishing and self-caring.

Perhaps you are at home with the need to create shorter chunks before choosing a practice to change state. Or you have to plan the way that you will do a particular task, maybe with some assistance. What you can do, what you want to do, and how you do it will vary enormously between people. You will carve out your own way forward, making sure that each day you are doing things that matter to you, even just for short periods (see Habits). Once you have done them, you can acknowledge your success—mark it in the sand. Many people find it useful to make notes (sometimes brief) in their journal each day, which is your log of wins that you can refer to and build upon.

2. Joy and pleasure

What brings joy and pleasure for you? Is it music? Reading? Being with loved ones and friends? Sitting in the garden? Building a model? So many things!

Are you doing any of them currently? Would you like to? Can you populate your day with moments of joy and pleasure? Yes!

Some people find it useful to make a list of the things that make them feel this way, lifting their energy. Then you can choose which to do when, and how. Perhaps you start by spending a few minutes, but then you can gradually build the time. As ever, you can acknowledge the feelings and the success.

3. Laughter

How often do you laugh? Really laugh? It is understandable that humour dries up when you are suffering. But what happens if you start to watch some things that would usually make you laugh? Perhaps you are willing to give it a try. Dose yourself on comedy moments throughout the day. There are plenty to be found on YouTube for instance.

Sometimes it can hurt when you laugh. But you know that you are not doing any harm, and overall the effect can be a positive one. As stated elsewhere, Norman Cousins who wrote 'An Anatomy of an Illness' essentially laughed himself better from an autoimmune disease that medicine was unable to help. I am not saying that you will recover by just laughing as this was his experience, but there is something distantly healthy that can happen. Share it with others and you will also gain the effects of sharing and bonding.

4. Contribution

Trying to move your attention (see Focus and attention) outwards towards something to someone else can have a positive impact on pain. I think this is more than a distraction, which is more of a momentary change of focus. If purposely you are attending to another's needs, then you are changing state with the intent to be useful and supportive. This is a healthy action and means that you will feel differently.

As with all the practices that seek to help you change state, the pain can come back into your attention. I am not suggesting that once you have moved away from feeling pain that is it. You will need to refocus. You may choose to use a practice such as RAIN discussed in the Challenging moments section. The more moments you can spend in good or better states, the better your day will be when you look back, especially if you end on a high (see below).

Examples of contributing could be listening to a loved one, helping your child do her homework, doing some household tasks (as best you can), or volunteering for an organisation. There are many ways depending on your skills, strengths, and existing situation that are viewed increasingly dynamically (i.e. it will change). For instance, you may start contributing in some small way but will be able to do more in time.

5. Appreciation (also see Gratitude)

It turns out that this is a skill of being well by the fact that you can practise appreciating other people as a way of being before you spend time with them. The quality of our relationships and the interactions within them have an impact on our health. I talk about this in more detail in the Building Health section.

You can also look around for other things that you can appreciate, including your own strengths. Often when suffering persistent pain, thoughts about the things you can't do predominate, frequently accompanied by the self-critic. This makes us feel bad. It is not necessarily an instant change, but by regularly looking out for things to appreciate, it becomes a habit, just as that of looking out for a painful world. As ever, there is no blame here. Instead, just gaining insight into how the human mind, how your mind works so that you can move forward in a better direction.

6. Finish on a high

Whatever we do, if we finish on a good note or a high, we tend to remember it as better than perhaps it was. Perhaps you went for a meal that turned out to be a very average main course (I could have cooked it better myself …), but the dessert was superb. Somehow this transforms the overall experience. We also reference the highs and lows throughout rather than the humdrum in between that makes up the bulk of our time. Just the highlights are noted, and the lowlights.

Bearing this in mind, maybe you can think of some ways to finish your day with a positive. For example, some people write down their successes at the end of the day, acknowledging their wins in preparation for the next day. Other people make sure they do all that they can to create the conditions for a restful night. Many struggle with sleep, so doing your best to cultivate a sleep habit is vital (see Sleep).

I hope from this section that you can see a way of living life to improve your life as opposed to waiting for a treatment of some kind to make you better. Why wait when you can get started now?

Encouragement points

- Focus on what you want rather than what you don't. In other words, focus on how to live your life better and better.

- Think about what matters to you in your life, and make decisions based on them.
- Make a list of things that bring you joy and pleasure. And do them each day.

Exercise

'If there was a magic pill for health, exercise would be it.' RS

'One rep is better than none!' RS

This kind of message is often out there, and it is true. But we need to be clear on what exercise is and how you can go about it in the right way for you. For some people, getting back to exercise or increasing their level of exercise is a major goal. For others, they know the importance of being active and moving (you may like to review the Movement section—'motion is lotion'). Often the issue is not knowing how to go about it. Let's clear that up.

Exercise is known for its wide-reaching benefits on your health. Research and people's experiences tell us that we feel better in ourselves, self-esteem and confidence build, we get fitter and stronger, concentration and focus improve, we buffer against many of the serious conditions such as heart disease and diabetes, and we are better able to deal with day-to-day living. Anecdotally, many people will talk about how exercise is an important part of their routine, building and maintaining their health, or as a way to deal with the harder aspects of life. For example, exercise is a key component of dealing with depression and anxiety.

And believe it or not, many people enjoy exercise! Maybe not always at the time …

But it sounds so simple!

Get exercising and you'll feel good. It's true in many cases, of course, but if you are suffering from chronic pain it can be a real challenge, even if you want to exercise. There can be a fear of moving and being active because of the pain. It can seem counterintuitive to be exercising if it causes more pain and suffering, especially if there is a belief that pain means injury. Understanding that this relationship is poor helps, but equally, to ignore the pain and push on through can lead to a bumpy ride.

Finding a way, your way, with exercise is an important part of shaping a positive future. Pleasingly, there are many forms, and if we all exercise with physical activity, you may discover some surprising things!

What is exercise?

You will have an idea about exercise through your own experiences. Perhaps it makes you think of school days in a good way, or maybe not. The word may evoke images of a gym, someone running or wearing particular clothing. So initially, exercise is whatever you think it is, which may or may not enthuse you.

By definition, exercise is 'a subset of physical activity that is planned, structured, and repetitive and has as a final or an intermediate objective the improvement or maintenance of physical fitness', where physical activity is defined as 'any bodily movement produced by skeletal muscles that results in energy expenditure' (Caspersen et al., 1985).

Being physically active includes not only exercising but also day-to-day activities such as walking, housework, playing with the kids, and gardening. Both exercising and physical activity usually have a purpose, which is useful. It could be to build wellness, but equally it could be to go shopping, mow the lawn, or hoover the lounge. Any activity above baseline has a benefit. Baseline means sedentary, essentially sitting and not moving.

With exercise being a form of physical activity, you can use the words that suit and motivate you. If the thought of exercise is off putting, but the idea of going for a walk appeals, then go for the second option. How you frame it to yourself will determine how encouraged you feel and hence the likelihood of following through.

It turns out that mindset and the way you think about exercise and activity makes a difference—knowing that you are being active and that this has a positive effect. In a study a few years ago, the authors discovered that telling female hotel attendants that their work met the recommendations for healthy activity levels resulted in changes in their weight, blood pressure, body fat, and body mass index (Crum & Langer, 2007).

What did the attendants change? Their perception versus those who were not given the same information. It appears there is a placebo effect when it comes to exercise. In other words, the way you think about what you are doing matters in objective, measurable ways. This is yet another example of how inseparable are the mind and body. There really is just one experience that we can shape in different ways.

Moving and exercising nourishes your body and changes the way you feel and think. Motion is lotion.

All experiences are underpinned by the biological state of your body as you now know. We don't have an explanation as to how the body state becomes a lived experience yet, but it is definitely happening. For example, it is known that muscles release chemicals known as myokines, including some that are anti-inflammatory. This is important in the face of being sedentary, which is pro-inflammatory. Inflammation plays a role in the loss of muscle mass and strength (sarcopenia) and the accumulation of visceral fat (Pratesi et al., 2013).

Many risk factors emerge from an inflammatory condition: diabetes, heart disease, depression, chronic pain, cancer, and dementia. Exercise and activity provide a powerful antidote, reducing the probabilities of these increasingly common problems that are so impacting upon quality of life.

Chunk it

To gain the benefits of exercise, you don't need to do it all at once. In fact, it may be better to have bouts of exercise, or movement and any specific techniques at different times throughout the day. The latter means you accumulate the gains from a range of practices. Much like you don't drink two litres of water in the morning and then have no more during the rest of the day. Instead you have drinks on a regular and consistent basis to maintain hydration—hopefully. You will notice that the words regular and consistent feature regularly and consistently!

In the Planning section, I spoke of how you can organise your day so that you are successful with tasks that need to be done, activities you want to do and the important rest breaks in between. Exercise or being active if you prefer, is interwoven into the day, occupying some of these chunks, to be acknowledged and ticked off as you go. You form a habit. A positive pattern.

Making it important

You can decide to make it important for you to be active in your own way. If being well and healthy is one of your values, then being active is the way. Equally, if family is important to you, then being well is also key, which in turn requires regular activity. Without the ability to be active and move, life is very restricted, as many people suffering from chronic pain know. So how can we become more active, gradually?

First, you may like to think about the answer to these questions:

- Why is it important for me to be active each day?
- What will life be like for me when I am more active? What will I be able to do?
- What will life be like if I don't practise being active?

Your start point

You have decided to create a new habit because your wellness is important to you or because family matters and you want to be able to participate and contribute. There may be other reasons.

Where do you start?

You need to establish your baseline. What are you able to do, however small? Remember, this is the starting point and not the end result. Look out for the parts of you that are not so encouraging! Try to work with the other parts of you that know the benefits and the gains you will make, acknowledging any voices that are critical but not feeding them.

Set the bar low to begin. What is definitely achievable? Not maybe or perhaps. Create the best conditions for a win that you can build on. And when you have been successful, acknowledge it. This is good journal material and something you can appreciate in yourself, the fact that you set a goal and followed through. Confidence and a sense of self-reliance notch up each time.

If this is a challenge for you, it will be important to seek advice. Having a conversation with a healthcare professional who knows how to prescribe exercise can be really helpful. It can be difficult and perhaps a little scary, however, you can be proud of what you achieve.

A routine

Creating a weekly and daily routine means that you know what you are doing and when. Written down in the diary or on a visible schedule makes it more likely you will follow through and be successful.

To gain the benefits of being active, you need repetition. Regular and consistent actions (your practice) are key, each one a step in the right direction. You have goals you are working towards, signposts along the way, yet the way continues indefinitely. This is a route of mastery. There is no end to living your best life. Like any peak performer or person at the top of their game, you continue to practise. And like cleaning your teeth … you wouldn't stop that habit because you have practised enough would you? Each time you practise, you are confirming that version of you.

I didn't follow my plan

Sometimes you miss a practice. Maybe something came up or you were tired after a bad night's sleep or feeling more pain. Perhaps you lacked motivation and the part of you encouraging staying in the chair won out.

It often feels bad.

We don't need to make it worse by continuing to berate ourselves.

You already know that you didn't practice. But the narrative can continue anyway, pointing it out and making other unhelpful comments.

This is when self-compassion is important. Being kind to yourself and trying to be understanding and encouraging. One way is to think about what you would say to someone you care about who finds themselves in the same position.

What would you say to them to encourage? Try saying this to yourself now, noticing how that feels. Sow the seed. These kinds of practices can feel a little strange to begin with, but then you realise that you are talking to yourself all the time anyway! That's not the issue. The issue is what you listen to, or not, and then what you do. Thoughts will come and there is nothing you can do to stop them directly—'I tried to clear my mind'; good luck! Instead you can be aware, such awareness cultivated through mindful practice (see Mindful section), notice and let the thoughts pass by. 'Hello old friend. I see you', said Thich Nhat Hanh, Zen master.

When you do practise, whatever happens, there is an opportunity to learn.

When you don't practise, there is an opportunity to learn. What stopped me? How can I better deal with this? Was there a circumstance out of my control? You will recall that there are always circumstances to consider. If you have slept badly and feel more pain and fatigue, this is not your fault. You have not chosen these experiences. Considering these circumstances, what is the best course of action? Perhaps to recover, use movement and breathing. A time may arise later that day when you feel better and are able to try some exercise, or the next day.

There is a need for flexibility in planning exercise and activity. Trying to progress according to a rigid plan of progression often leads to more pain and suffering as it assumes a linear recovery. There is nothing linear about getting better as you know. So, you need a way of moving forward that is adaptable, in step with the reality of the unpredictable, uncertain, and varied life that is the case for all humans. The expectation that there is a straight and smooth road ahead causes many problems for people. Although it is an attractive prospect, when you study your own life, you see the reality. Daily mindful practice helps with this realisation.

You are doing your best.

Accumulation of benefits

Over the day you will accumulate steps and movements. It can add up without you realising. If fatigue is a feature of your lived experience, keeping a note of what you are doing is important. Planning and periodising your day is a practical way of doing this more accurately. It is unlikely to be perfect, but again, you are doing your best to account for what you are doing.

If there is something you need to do on a given day that you know will require a good level of energy, then you may plan your time differently. It could be that this is your form of exercise for the day. This is part of being flexible and planning accordingly.

Progressing

There will be a point when you feel that your existing level of activity has become easier. You sense that you could try a little more. This comes off the back of consistent practice at a certain level. The regularity leads to an organic progression without pushing.

This is different from a set progression when each week you add time or distance, regardless of how you feel. I suggest that instead, you check in to see how you are and then set your expectations accordingly. This way you are working with yourself, and importantly setting your expectations more in line with reality, which gets better results (see Expectations).

Progression and growth are normal human experiences. Clearly you can also get stuck (e.g. pain, depression, anxiety, addiction). But you can also get unstuck, which is what you are doing right now as you read this and update your understanding and open the range of possibilities for positive action.

By working within your window of tolerance, organically your activity levels will expand. That is what happens because you have created evidence of what you can do that is better, which forms predictions for the next time. What you do now informs what will come. This is an important principle to consider with all your activities.

You are not where you want to be, yet. The key three-letter word. You are working towards something, but from where you are now. This is acceptance and an openness to reality that may differ from your narrative, allowing you the freedom to progress.

I am active

Thinking of yourself as someone who is active helps make those decisions. If this is how you see yourself, an active version (in your own way), then you will find it easier to step into those shoes.

'I am the kind of person who is active.'

This is how you see yourself and then step into those shoes. Then take it step by step.

Exercise and pain

One of the reasons activity levels drop is because of pain. After an injury, this is useful because it allows the body to heal, although movement is important for tissue recovery. If pain persists, it can still feel as if you should be resting and protecting yourself despite the fact that you do need some movement and activity. In time it can get harder and harder—a downward spiral.

Some people try to keep going and push on with mixed results, but usually dominated by pain. Others take it easy until they feel better, and then go for it. Overdoing it then causes a spike in the pain and the need to slow down again. This is called the over-under activity cycle that makes it very difficult to progress in any meaningful way. It is stop-start and can be disheartening at times.

A better way is to be consistent and regular starting with a low baseline as described above. Whilst there are still ups and downs, the ride is smoother and more encouraging. Plus you learn skills to surf the waves, and to get back onto your board when you are thrown off.

Feeling pain after exercising is normal. Most people have had the experience of waking up the day after doing a new or different activity feeling stiff and sore. This is often welcomed as a sign of achievement. Perhaps a badge of honour.

In persistent pain states, however, feeling pain is usually deemed to indicate something bad or negative, something gone wrong, or a worry about the risk of re-injury. In most cases this is unlikely. Check what you have been doing. What actually happened? What is actually happening now? Did you really make a bad choice to exercise, or did you just not get the result you expected or wanted? When things don't turn out the way you want, it does not make it a bad decision. Often it was a good one. Moving and exercising is typically a good idea. The key now that whatever has happened has happened, is to think about what you can learn. What will you do differently but in line with your picture of success? Avoidance is not in line with your picture of success of course.

So, unlikely to be an injury (if you are really unsure, check with your health-care professional), you can remind yourself that because of prior experiences of pain during or after exercise, it continues to be the best explanation for what is happening in your lived world. Your body systems expect a painful world and so that is what you are more likely to experience, until there is new evidence to suggest something else; e.g. getting better, a good experience.

It is also useful to know that movement plays a part in recovery and healing from an injury. There is rarely a reason not to move in some way.

Being active and increasing your tolerance for day-to-day living is a vital part of getting better. It often takes courage, especially if fear of movement (kinesiophobia) has set in. This happens over a period of time when you repeatedly suffer the pain associated with moving (a worse-than-expected outcome) until you begin to anticipate pain beforehand. We know that the more you anticipate something will hurt, the more it does. This is why understanding your pain together with creating better and good experiences (see below) is a way forward.

'Understanding your pain helps you engage in the activities you want to do, and build confidence.' RS

It is likely that you will feel some pain when you are being active or afterwards. When you know and expect this as the norm, plus have ways to think and deal with it, you can feel more confident in what you are doing. Having more confidence and know-how actually changes the experience of what it is like. People tell me that they did experience some pain, but that they could manage it and on balance enjoy the activity. This is an important step as you are actively creating evidence that things can be better for you.

Fear of pain can be driven by different thoughts. Some people fear that they are re-injuring themselves, but when they understand their pain, realise this is not the case with day-to-day activities and exercises. Others fear the pain itself because of its intensity and impact. Again, understanding your pain helps to address the fears, and many people are able to overcome them and feel a sense of achievement. You can deal with your fear of pain if it is a barrier. If you are really struggling with this aspect, I recommend working with a chronic pain specialist or as I call it, a Pain Coach.

Following the guidelines suggested here will help you to maintain your programme and progress.

Having good experiences

Setting up active situations when you do as well as, or better than, expected is what can help you to recover your ability to be active over time. Being present and noticing how you are doing helps to gather the evidence that you can and will shape a positive future.

I encourage people to work within their window of tolerance. This means that on balance, the chosen activity can be thought of as a positive experience. There may have been some pain and symptoms, but they were manageable and the focus was on the activity.

If you set out to have a good experience by setting the goals at the right level, you are maximising the chances of this happening. In other words, match your expectations with reality as closely as you can.

For example, you expect to be able to walk for thirty minutes. Part of you says that is what you should be able to do, based on prior experiences. If the reality is that you are able to walk fifteen minutes, there is a clear mismatch. If you bring your expectations in line and accept that fifteen minutes is the goal, then they will meet and you have a good experience (despite a self-critic that needs managing). If you do not bring them into alignment, it feels bad because you do worse than expected. This kind of repeating cycle is thought to underpin a shift towards becoming stuck with pain as a repeated prediction. Alternatively, you may decide to push on to thirty minutes anyway and then find that you suffer more pain later. Again, worse than expected.

Having repeated good and better experiences as best you can by planning and prioritising, helps you move towards your picture of success.

Interweaving activity into your day

You know that you can chunk your exercises, movements, and activities through the day to get jobs done (being useful) and to gain the positive effects (wellness). A household chore can be thought of as an exercise. Consider that it is well thought out that varied and functional movements are good for us, which is why some people choose training that includes crawling, climbing, jumping, and other skills. This may not be appropriate for you, but just to illustrate the point that exercise comes in many forms. If it so happens that you empty the dishwasher, carry some clothes upstairs, or walk to work, you are also doing something meaningful. More on this in the Movement section and the motion is lotion strategy.

You may like to think about how you can bring movement and exercise into your daily routine. For example, you practice balancing whilst the kettle boils, you do a few squats when you first stand up from being at your desk, or a few calf raises before you sit down to watch a film. Of course, at other times, you have planned other exercises that are part of your programme.

Remember that one rep is better than none and brings benefits over not having moved.

Specific exercises and training

With certain conditions or situations, you will need specific exercises. For instance, you may need to train your body position sense. This is knowing where you are in space, which you wouldn't normally think about. However, when you are suffering persistent pain, your body sense and movement can change, adapting to enable you to keep going, but at a cost. On a practical level, you may have noticed being clumsy, or bumping into furniture, making misjudgements, or finding it hard to move with ease.

Body sense, or proprioception to give it the scientific name, is often trained with balance exercises if it relates to the whole body. If you are trying to develop more efficient arm or hand movements, you will use visual feedback as you make gentle corrections whilst practising a given task such as picking up small items, or using a keyboard.

There are benefits from strength and mobility exercises. These must be prescribed, starting with a low baseline so you are following the principle of curating good experiences to build upon. Your healthcare professional should be able to help you design this element of your programme, choosing the reps and sets, plus of course recovery time. There must be flexibility built into your programme as each time you practice is a new time. The number of reps may vary. I tend to give people a range to work to and encourage a check-in beforehand, then estimate the number you will do.

The goal is to be active and successful from doing so in a way that can be thought of as a good experience. The goal is not to complete a certain number of reps. Remember process over prize as a principle.

Rest and recovery

After a bout of exercise or activity, it is vital to allow your body to adapt by giving yourself a period of rest and recharge to recover. Depending on what you have done, you will decide for how long and what you do. Whatever it is, try to be consistent and make this part of your exercise habit.

Recovery time is as important as the activity itself for adaptation. You only need to look at professional athletes' training programmes to understand this. The greatest recovery happens when you sleep, so if your bedtime is disrupted, making sure you have time during the day is critical. Also, working on your sleep pattern is important for this reason and others that pertain to your well-being.

If you have been exercising, a good half hour to an hour of minimal activity to allow your body systems to return to baseline is advisable. There will be variability from person to person. If you monitor yourself, you will be able to make better judgements in order to meet your needs.

In the Pauses section, I spoke of the necessity to stop and check in between activities so we don't bring the energy of the previous task to the one you are doing now. Noticing how you are and choosing a practice that is nurturing or useful means you are on track. Recovery after exercise is an extended pause.

The types of things that you can do to recover include driving water, eating a snack, breathing practice, resting with your feet up, sitting and reading, doing something that relaxes you that does not use much energy such as listening to an audiobook or music, or watching TV. You might also include a few stretches (I often call this lengthening) if you find them helpful.

Encouragement points

- Exercise and being active have many health benefits and should be an integral part of getting better.
- You can choose the types of exercises and activities that you enjoy, and perhaps try something new.
- You need to set your baseline low and build flexibly.
- Try to match your expectations with reality when setting a goal.
- Interweave activity and movement into your day, including any specific cxcrciscs.
- Fear of pain must be addressed.
- Rest and recovery is a part of building wellness as much as the exercise.

Impermanence

'Insights are the catalysts of positive change. Impermanence is one such insight.' RS

'Thanks to impermanence, everything is possible.' Thich Nhat Hanh

You may be wondering why I end on an insight. There are many that can be useful. Maybe you have your own. Elsewhere I have encouraged you to find phrases or mantras that help you stay on your path.

Insights are the catalysts of positive change. What I mean by this is that when an insight becomes apparent, the world shifts and changes. Realising something like impermanence changes the way you think and do things; for the better! Together with the insight that it is not what is happening as much as how you relate to it, impermanence is one of the most potent catalysts.

Impermanence is one of the three dharma seals, together with no-self and nirvana. Insight into these, Buddhism argues, is the way we touch reality. Others also noticed that no moment is ever the same. Heraclitus spoke of never bathing in the same river and Confucius observed how the river always flows. It is the same with life and our experiences, despite how they might appear to us.

'Thanks to impermanence, everything is possible', said Thich Nhat Hanh, the father and teacher of engaged Buddhism who died the week I am writing these words. An influence upon me and my work for over 30 years, Thich Nhat Hanh, shared his compassion and teachings to promote peaceful, social change.

Life is only possible because things are changing all the time. No moment is ever the same. No pain experience can ever be the same, however it appears to us. If you look closely, you will notice that what can stay the same is the narrative, although even that is impermanent. The words can be the same words, but delivered to yourself or another person in a different moment makes them fundamentally different as well. You may be wondering why this is important.

Firstly because this is the nature of things and the closer we are to reality, the better we can navigate the world and live well. Secondly, the fact that whatever is happening will change means that suffering can change. In other words, we can ease our suffering, which is one of the Four Noble Truths. The others are that in life there is suffering, there are causes of suffering and that there is a path that leads to the end of suffering.

When you are having a difficult time, remember that no matter how you feel, it will pass, can be helpful. It is a form of self-soothing or self-coaching, reminding yourself of a positive future to come. In doing so, you also create some space to think a little more clearly. In this space, it is more likely to occur to you that there are other practices you can use to ease your suffering.

For example, coming back to your breathing, which is a way of applying the brakes further. It does take practice to become more skilful at doing this, typically when you can concentrate, so at easier times (see Breathing) and as a day-to-day habit. Each practice you get a little better, meaning that when you need to use it, it becomes more effective.

Meditation practice helps you to realise impermanence. As you sit and practise, you will notice how things are constantly changing for you. Thoughts and feelings come and go. Sensations come and go. Sounds and what you see appear and then pass by as each moment goes by and your attention moves. You often start to notice how all our perceptions appear in our awareness without actually doing anything. In other words, there's nothing you actually have to do for your experience of you to exist. There is a complex dynamic at play that you can notice and let be in your awareness, bringing about the transformation of experiences such as pain.

This is a powerful insight and becomes transformative in terms of being in touch with reality rather than being whisked away by thoughts about the past or future, and getting caught up in it all, far from what is actually happening in your world. You will read more in the Mindfulness section.

Encouragement points

- Life is only possible because of impermanence.
- Things are always changing, despite how it feels or what you tell yourself.
- Practicing mindfulness helps you gain this insight.

Section 7   Bringing it all together

'Now is the only time. You shape your future by the decision and action you take now and keep taking.' RS

Now that you have read through the practices, tools, strategies, and exercises, we can look at how you create your own programme based upon your needs.

At this point, if you are working with a healthcare professional, you may like to discuss with them how you can integrate this programme with any other work you are doing. Are there particular practices or tools that you want to try?

The overarching aim must always be the steps to take to achieve your picture of success. Re-clarifying this may be useful at this point.

My picture(s) of success:

*
*
*

Your picture of success gives you direction and a reference point: what can I do right now that takes me towards my picture of success? Am I taking steps in line with where I want to go? It is helpful and motivating to remember why it matters to you.

My picture(s) of success matter because:

*
*
*

Which tools and practices resonated?

As you were reading through the tools and practices section, which ones brought up a positive feeling? Perhaps you have been trying some of them. You may have sensed that these particular activities meet your needs.

Were there any that you were unsure about? There will be a reason. Looking into why this is the case can be revealing. It may be a challenging area or questions an existing belief. This does not mean the practice will not be useful for you. Examining why you feel unsure can reveal whether there is a good reason. Bringing this flexibility into your thinking is very healthy. Many of your beliefs are long-held, but what is the evidence?

Instead of accepting your belief as a given, you can think like a scientist and view your ideas and opinions as a hypothesis. The more resistance you feel, the more you realise you are attached to the idea. Being curious about both the idea and why you might be holding on so tight can be revealing.

There is nothing wrong with being wrong! Updating your beliefs is learning, which is the essence of overcoming pain. You know that your beliefs are playing a role in your actual pain experience. If your pain is sticky, which is probably the reason you are reading this book, there is a stuckness in your belief system that is not updating. Getting flexibility back into the systems is key to moving forward, so this becomes an opportunity to do that.

Creating your individual programme

My hope is that you will take the philosophy and shape it into your own as you design your way onwards. The Planning section guides you on making the framework, filled by the content of the practices, exercises, and tools—your habits that build on existing ones that work.

There are four themes you can use as a framework (see below). These are the things you can control and work upon day to day towards your pictures of success. It is a journey of learning and growth, a process that started well before the moment you first noted pain and is shaped by the socioeconomic environment, past experiences, beliefs, and expectations. Taking a pain experience out as a separate entity for 'treatment' is not the reality.

The way you and your body systems respond to suffering was learned in childhood and taken into adulthood. It has taken your whole life to reach this very moment when you are reading and responding to these words. What you are feeling when you are in pain, is the sum of all those responses that have been learned. The key question is whether these responses are working or not? Are you moving forward or are you stuck?

The four interrelated themes:

1. Specific skills and strategies: the practical steps you take towards all your specific goals throughout each day.
2. Skills and strategies to live your best life: you are making decisions all day about what to do, what not to do, and how to do it. Clarity of thought and presence helps make the best choices in the moment, which comes from practices such as meditation and taking pauses. There are many examples of ways to go about being active and re-engaging with life throughout the book. This takes the bulk of your time (how many hours are you awake each day?), so thinking about how you will go about living, considering your current but ever-changing circumstances, will help you stay on your path. In so doing, you are aligning your expectations and reality, which matters for getting better.
3. Skills of being well: the daily pillars or habits that you put in place to build and sustain wellness. There are more obvious ones such as diet, prioritising sleep, and being active (eat, rest, move). Others that are important according to research are being able to pay attention, pursuing a purpose, connecting healthily with others (relationships; underpinned by awareness and communication), self-compassion, and resilience. The skills of being well can include and also enhanced by meditation practices, breathing exercises, and the ability to relax and create inner calm.
4. Skilful response to challenging moments: what is happening is what is happening. How you relate to it and respond is what matters because this is what you can do, and makes it what it is. Knowing that you can update your responses and then having a range of choices gives you the flexibility to roll with situations and be able to let go. This is at the heart of easing your own suffering. This is also the opportunity to learn: does the way I am responding work or not?

There is overlap between these themes, with some practices being useful for more than one. For example, a breathing awareness practice is a great way to bring calm and presence to your day and a way to deal with your own suffering. As you know, to transform our suffering, we must be present rather than try to avoid it or run away, which achieves nothing. This can feel alien to many people, especially in the West where we are not trained how to suffer.

This may sound unusual. But in other cultures and philosophies, learning how to suffer as a way to ease suffering is part of day-to-day being. Suffering is seen as very much a part of life to be accepted, together with the fact that we can ease our own suffering by learning about the truth of things. This is the essence of mindful practice.

You do not need to incorporate all of the practices and tools. In fact, this would be impossible! You would be doing nothing else. Remember that the most important principle is to live life in the best way that you can, filling your time with meaningful, useful, and important activities. This often means gradually reconnecting with people, purpose and the planet, building up over time (at the right pace for you), surfing the ups and downs as best you can, knowing that things are always changing and you are in the driving seat.

In my work with people suffering chronic pain and in this book I have turned the model on its head. Instead of waiting for pain to get better to start living, you start living as a way to get better and overcome pain. You fill your life with more and more meaning in what you are doing, whilst building your health and using specific practices to meet your needs and relate and respond skilfully to the challenging movements as learning opportunities. Much of this is about you self-caring and practicing self-compassion as you create the conditions for a positive future.

Writing out your programme

When you write out your programme it is visible to you and a reminder. You can also tick off as you go, acknowledging your wins along the way. It makes it more likely that you will follow through and take positive action if you have a hard copy.

Some people create a colour-coded diary. This means that you can glance at your schedule and notice whether you have your activities and recharge time balanced. You may choose colours for work, exercise, particular practices, rest time, joyful activities, and family time for instance. If you see that a category is missing, you can adjust your schedule.

Building on existing habits

You may have some habits and practices that are working for you. These you can keep going as you bring in new choices. What got you here, won't get you there is a phrase worth bearing in mind. In other words, it is important to be reviewing your programme and practices periodically. This will give you the chance to see what is continuing to deliver results and where you may need to update or progress what you are doing.

Essentially you are building on what works for you.

I wish you well.

Encouragement points

- Now you can design your individualised, holistic programme by choosing the practices and tools that meet your needs.
- Build on what is already going well.
- Write out your schedule for the week so that you can follow and tick off.
- Colour coding can give you a quick view on the balance of your week.
- Review your programme periodically to make sure that you are heading in the right direction.

References

Ackerley, R.D., Wasling, H.D., Liljencrantz, J.D., Olausson, H.D., Johnson, R.D. et al. (2014). Human C-tactile afferents are tuned to the temperature of a skin-stroking caress. *J Neurosci.* 34:2879–2883.

Aiyegbusi, O.L., Hughes, S.E., Turner, G., Rivera, S.C., McMullan, C., Chandan, J.S., Haroon, S., Price, G., Davies, E.H., Nirantharakumar, K., Sapey, E., & Calvert, M.J. (2021). TLC study group. Symptoms, complications and management of long COVID: A review. *J R Soc Med.* Sep;114(9):428–442.

Alshelh, Z. et al. (2022). Neuroimmune signatures in chronic low back pain subtypes. *Brain* 145(3):1098–1110.

Baliki, M.N., Petre, B., Torbey, S., Herrmann, K.M., Huang, L., Schnitzer, T.J., Fields, H.L., & Apkarian, A.V. (2012). Corticostriatal functional connectivity predicts transition to chronic back pain. *Nat Neurosci.* Jul 1;15(8):1117–1119.

Bauer, M.E., & Teixeira, A.L. (2019). Inflammation in psychiatric disorders: What comes first? *Ann NY Acad Sci.* 1437:57–67.

Berenbaum, F. (2013). Osteoarthritis as an inflammatory disease (osteoarthritis is not osteoarthrosis!). *Osteoarthritis Cartilage.* Jan;21(1):16–21.

Beurel, E., Toups, M., & Nemeroff, C.B. (2020). The bidirectional relationship of depression and inflammation: Double trouble. *Neuron.* Jul 22;107(2):234–256.

Bonanno, G. (2021). *The End of Trauma.* Basic Books.

Brown, D. TED talk: Mentalism, mind reading and the art of getting inside your head. https://www.ted.com/talks/derren_brown_mentalism_mind_reading_and_the_art_of_getting_inside_your_head

Carel, H. (2008). *Illness (The Art of Living Series).* Routledge.

Carragee, E.J., Alamin, T.F., Miller, J.L., & Carragee, J.M. (2005). Discographic, MRI and psychosocial determinants of low back pain disability and remission: A prospective study in subjects with benign persistent back pain. *Spine J.* 5(1):24–35.

Caspersen, C.J., Powell, K.E., & Christenson, G.M. (1985). Physical activity, exercise, and physical fitness: Definitions and distinctions for health-related research. *Public Health Rep.* Mar–Apr;100(2):126–131.

Chödrön, P. https://www.lionsroar.com/how-we-get-hooked-shenpa-and-how-we-get-unhooked/

Ciaunica, A., & Charlton, J. (2018). When the self slips: What depersonalization can say about the self. Aeon. https://aeon.co/essays/what-can-depersonalisation-disorder-say-about-the-self

Ciaunica, A., Shmeleva, E.V., & Levin, M. (2023). The brain is not mental! coupling neuronal and immune cellular processing in human organisms. *Front Integr Neurosci.* May 17;17:1057622.

Clark, A. (2016). *Surfing Uncertainty: Prediction, Action, and the Embodied Mind.* OUP.

Clark, A. (2023). *The Experience Machine.* Penguin.

Cole, S.W., Hawkley, L.C., Arevalo, J.M., Sung, C.Y., Rose, R.M., Cacioppo, J.T. (2007). Social regulation of gene expression in human leukocytes. *Genome Biol.* 8(9):R189.

Cooperrider, D. https://www.davidcooperrider.com/ai-process/

Cousins, N. (2005). *Anatomy of an Illness: As Perceived by the Patient.* Ed: Twentieth Anniversary. W. W. Norton & Company.

Crum, A.J., & Langer, E.J. (2007). Mind-set matters: Exercise and the placebo effect. *Psychol Sci.* Feb;18(2):165–171.

Dahl, C.J., Wilson-Medenhall, C.D., & Davidson, R.J. (2020). The plasticity of well-being: A training-based framework for the cultivation of human flourishing. *PNAS* 117(51):32197–32206.

Daniels, T., Olsen, E., & Tyrka, A.R. (2020). Stress and psychiatric disorders: The role of mitochondria. *Annu Rev Clin Psychol.* May 07;16:165–186.

Dantzer, R., O'Connor, J.C., Freund, G.G., Johnson, R.W., & Kelley, K.W. (2008). From inflammation to sickness and depression: When the immune system subjugates the brain. *Nat Rev Neurosci.* Jan;9(1):46–56.

De Haan, S. (2020). *Enactive Psychiatry.* Cambridge: Cambridge University Press.

Diego, M.A., Field, T. (2009). Moderate pressure massage elicits a parasympathetic nervous system response. *Int J Neurosci.* 119(5):630–638.

Dum, R.P., Levinthal, D.J., & Strick, P.L. (2019). The mind–body problem: Circuits that link the cerebral cortex to the adrenal medulla. *PNAS* 116(52):26321–26328.

Emmons, R. (2020). Why Gratitude Is Good. Greater Good Magazine, November 16. https://greatergood.berkeley.edu/article/item/why_gratitude_is_good

Engel, G.L. (1977). The need for a new medical model: A challenge for biomedicine. *Science* Apr 8;196(4286):129–136.

Engel, G.L. (1980). The clinical application of the biopsychosocial model. *Am J Psychiatry.* May;137(5):535–544.

Epstein, M. (2022). *The Zen of Therapy: Uncovering a Hidden Kindness in Life.* Penguin Press.

Ericsson, K.A. & Harwell, K.W. (2019). Deliberate practice and proposed limits on the effects of practice on the acquisition of expert performance: Why the original definition matters and recommendations for future research. *Front. Psychol., Sec. Educational Psychology* 10.

Ericsson, K.A., Krampe, R.T., & Tesch-Romer, C. (1993). The role of deliberate practice in the acquisition of expert performance. *Psychol Rev.* 100(3):363–406.

Ericsson, K.A., & Kyle, H.W. (2019). Deliberate practice and proposed limits on the effects of practice on the acquisition of expert performance: Why the original definition matters and recommendations for future research. *Front. Psychol.* Oct 25;2396:1–19.

Espie, C.A. (2022). The '5 principles' of good sleep health. *J Sleep Res.* 31:e13502.

Feldman-Barrett, L. (2021). *Seven and a Half Lessons About the Brain.* Picador.

Ferreira, M.L. et al. (2023). Global, regional, and national burden of low back pain, 1990–2020, its attributable risk factors, and projections to 2050: A systematic analysis of the Global Burden of Disease Study 2021. *Lancet Rheumatol.* 5(6):E316–E329.

Fox, G.R., Kaplan, J., Damasio, H., & Damasio, A. (2015). Neural correlates of gratitude. *Front Psychol.* Sep 30;6:1491.

Garfinkel, S.N., Minati, L., Gray, M.A., Seth, A.K., Dolan, R.J., & Critchley, H.D. (2014). Fear from the heart: Sensitivity to fear stimuli depends on individual heartbeats. *J Neurosci.* May 7;34(19):6573–6582.

Ghaemi, S.N. (2020). Digital depression: A new disease of the millennium? *Acta Psych Scand.* 141(4):356–361.

Gifford, L. (1998). Pain, the tissues and the nervous system. *Physiotherapy* 84(1):127–136.

Gifford, L. https://giffordsachesandpains.com/

Gilbert, P. (2010). *Compassion Focused Therapy*. Routledge.

Gilbert, P. (2014). The origins and nature of compassion focused therapy. *Br J Clin Psychol.* 53:6–41.

Goldberg, D.S., & McGee, S.J. (2011). Pain as a global public health priority. *BMC Public Health.* Oct 6;11:770.

Goldberg, Y.P. et al. (2007). Loss-of-function mutations in the Nav1.7 gene underlie congenital indifference to pain in multiple human populations. *Clin Genetics.* 71(4):311–319.

Goldstein, P., Weissman-Fogel, I., Dumas, G., & Shamay-Tsoory, S.G. (2018). Brain-to-brain coupling during handholding is associated with pain reduction. *Proc Natl Acad Sci.* Feb 26;115(11):E2528–E2537.

Gottlieb, G. (1976). Conceptions of prenatal development: Behavioral embryology. *Psychological Review* 83:215–234.

Grace, P.M., Hutchinson, M.R., Maier, S.F., & Watkins, L.R. (2014). Pathological pain and the neuroimmune interface. *Nat Rev Immunol.* Apr;14(4):217–231.

Grady, C.L., Rieck, J.R., Nichol, D., Rodrigue, K.M., & Kennedy, K.M. (2020). Influence of sample size and analytic approach on stability and interpretation of brain-behavior correlations in task-related fMRI data. *Human Brain Mapp.* 42(1):204–219.

Henning, M., Fox, G.R., Kaplan, J., Damasio, H., & Damasio, A. (2017). A potential role for mu-opioids in mediating the positive effects of gratitude. *Front Psychol.* June 21;868:1–6..

Hoffman, K.M., Trawalter, S., Axt, J.R., & Oliver, M.N. (2016). Racial bias in pain assessment and treatment recommendations, and false beliefs about biological differences between blacks and whites. *Proc Natl Acad Sci.* Apr 19;113(16):4296–4301.

Iacobucci, G. (2022). Most black people in UK face discrimination from healthcare staff, survey finds. *BMJ* 378:o2337.

Ian Sample. 2019. 'War on cancer' metaphors may do harm, research shows. *The Guardian* Sat 10 Aug.

IASP. (2020). https://www.iasp-pain.org/publications/iasp-news/iasp-announces-revised -definition-of-pain/

Jackson, G. (2019). *Pain and Prejudice: A Call to Arms for Women and Their Bodies* (p. 360). Sydney: Allen & Unwin. ISBN: 9 7817 6052 9093.

Jain, S. (2020). Let's stop talking about "battling cancer". *Sci Am.* Jan.

Jepma, M., Koban, L., van Doorn, J., Jones, M., & Wager, T.D. (2018). Behavioural and neural evidence for self-reinforcing expectancy effects on pain. *Nat Hum Behav.* Nov;2(11):838–855.

Kabat-Zinn, J. (2023). *Mindfulness Meditation for Pain Relief: Practices to Reclaim Your Body and Your Life.* Sounds True.

Karns, C.M., Moore, W.E., & Mayr, U. (2017). The cultivation of pure altruism via gratitude: A functional MRI study of change with gratitude practice. *Front Hum Neurosci.* Dec 12; 599:1–14.

Kasch, R. et al. (2022). Association of Lumbar MRI findings with current and future back pain in a population-based cohort study. *Spine* 47(3):201–211.

Kasch, R., Truthmann, J., Hancock, M.J., Maher, C.G., Otto, M., Nell, C., Reichwein, N., Bülow, R., Chenot, J.F., Hofer, A., Wassilew, G., & Schmidt, C.O. (2022). Association of Lumbar MRI findings with current and future back pain in a population-based cohort study. *Spine (Phila Pa 1976)*. Feb 1;47(3):201–211.

Killingsworth, M.A., & Gilbert, D.T. (2010). A wandering mind is an unhappy mind. *Science*. Nov 12;330(6006):932.

Kiverstein, J., Kirchhoff, M.D., & Thacker, M. (2022). An embodied predictive processing theory of pain experience. *Rev Phil Psych*. 13:973–998.

Kline, C.E. (2014). The bidirectional relationship between exercise and sleep: Implications for exercise adherence and sleep improvement. *Am J Lifestyle Med*. Nov–Dec;8(6):375–379.

König, R.S., Albrich, W.C., Kahlert, C.R., Bahr, L.S., Löber, U., Vernazza, P., Scheibenbogen, C., & Forslund, S.K. (2022). The gut microbiome in Myalgic Encephalomyelitis (ME)/ Chronic Fatigue Syndrome (CFS). *Front Immunol*. Jan 3;12:628741.

Kristen Neff: https://self-compassion.org/

Kross, E. (2022). *Chatter: The Voice in Our Head and How to Harness It*. Vermilion.

Lakein, A. (1984). *How to Get Control of Your Time & Life*. Penguin Books Ltd.

Legrain, V., Iannetti, G.D., Plaghki, L., & Mouraux, A. (2011). The pain matrix reloaded: A salience detection system for the body. *Prog in Neurobiol*. 93(1):111–124.

Li, Q. (2010). Effect of forest bathing trips on human immune function. *Environ Health Prev Med*. Jan;15(1):9–17.

Li, Q., Nakadai, A., Matsushima, H., Miyazaki, Y., Krensky, A.M., Kawada, T., Morimoto, K. (2006). Phytoncides (wood essential oils) induce human natural killer cell activity. *Immunopharmacol Immunotoxicol*. 28(2):319–333.

Löken, L.S., Wessberg, J., Morrison, I., McGlone, F., & Olausson, H. (2009). Coding of pleasant touch by unmyelinated afferents in humans. *Nat Neurosci*. May;12(5):547–548.

Macchia, L. (2022). Pain trends and pain growth disparities, 2009–2021. *Econ Hum Biol*. Dec;47:101200.

Malys, M.K., & Mondelli, V. (2022). Could anti-inflammatory interventions earlier in development confer primary prevention of psychiatric disorders? *Harv Rev Psychiatry*. Jan–Feb 01;30(1):4–7.

Mansour, A.R., Farmer, M.A., Baliki, M.N., & Apkarian, A.V. (2014). Chronic pain: The role of learning and brain plasticity. *Restor Neurol Neurosci*. 32(1):129–139.

McCaffery, M. (1968). *Nursing Practice Theories Related to Cognition, Bodily Pain, and Man-Environment Interactions*. Los Angeles: University of California.

McNerney, S. (2011). A brief guide to embodied cognition: Why you are not your brain. *Sci Am*. Nov.

McWilliams, D.F., Dawson, O., Young, A., Kiely, P.D.W., Ferguson, E., & Walsh, D.A. (2019). Discrete trajectories of resolving and persistent pain in people with rheumatoid arthritis despite undergoing treatment for inflammation: Results from three UK cohorts. *J Pain*. Jun;20(6):716–727.

Meghani, S.H., Byun, E., & Gallagher, R.M. (2012). Time to take stock: A meta-analysis and systematic review of analgesic treatment disparities for pain in the United States. *Pain Med*. Feb;13(2):150–174.

Meints, S.M., Cortes, A., Morais, C.A., & Edwards, R.R. (2019). Racial and ethnic differences in the experience and treatment of noncancer pain. *Pain Manag*. May;9(3):317–334.

Melzack, R. (2001). Pain and the neuromatrix in the brain. *J Dent Educ*. 65(12):1378–1382.

Melzack, R., & Wall, P.D. (1965). Pain mechanisms: A new theory. *Science* 150:971–979.

Miller, W.R., & Moyers, T.B. (2021). *Effective Psychotherapists: Clinical Skills That Improve Client Outcomes*. Guildford Press.

Morris, G., & Maes, M. (2014). Mitochondrial dysfunctions in myalgic encephalomyelitis/chronic fatigue syndrome explained by activated immuno-inflammatory, oxidative and nitrosative stress pathways. *Metab Brain Dis*. Mar;29(1):19–36.

Nave, K., Deane, G., Miller, M. et al. (2022). Expecting some action: Predictive Processing and the construction of conscious experience. *Rev Phil Psych*. 13:1019–1037.

Nave, K., Deane, G., Miller, M., & Clark, A. (2020). Wilding the predictive brain. *WIREs Cogn Sci*. 11:e1542.

Newport, C. (2016). *Deep Work: Rules for Focused Success in a Distracted World*. Piatkus.

Nöe, A. (2004). *Action in Perception*. The MIT Press.

Pegg, M. (2012). *The Art of Strengths Coaching: The Complete Guide*. Management Books 2000 Ltd.

Plinsinga, M.L., Coombes, B.K., Mellor, R., Nicolson, P., Grimaldi, A., Hodges, P., Bennell, K., & Vicenzino, B. (2018). Psychological factors not strength deficits are associated with severity of gluteal tendinopathy: A cross-sectional study. *Eur J Pain*. 22(6):1124–1133.

Plum Village app: https://plumvillage.app/

Pratesi, A., Tarantini, F., & Di Bari, M. (2013). Skeletal muscle: An endocrine organ. *Clin Cases Miner Bone Metab*. Jan;10(1):11–14.

Rath, T. (2013). *Eat, Move, Sleep*. Missionday.

Rebecca Boehme Steven Hauser, Gregory J. Gerling Håkan Olausson. (2019). Distinction of self-produced touch and social touch at cortical and spinal cord levels. *PNAS* January 22;116(6):2290–2299.

Rice, A.S.C., Smith, B.H., & Blyth, F.M. (2016). Pain and the global burden of disease. *Pain* 157(4):791–796.

Robson, D. (2022). *The Expectation Effect: How Your Mindset can Transform your Life*. Canongate Books.

Rollnick, S., Miller, W.R., & Butler, C.C. (2022). *Motivational Interviewing in Health Care: Second Edition*. Guilford Press.

Sample, I. (2019). 'War on cancer' metaphors may do harm, research shows. *The Guardian*. Saturday Aug 10.

Sapolsky, R. (2004). *Why Zebras Don't Get Ulcers*. Holt Paperbacks.

Sapolsky, R. (2004). *Why Zebras Don't Get Ulcers: The Acclaimed Guide to Stress, Stress-Related Diseases, and Coping*. St. Martins Press, Revised and Upd edition.

Seth, A. (2021). *Being You: A New Science of Consciousness*. Faber & Faber.

Seth, A. TED Talk: Your brain hallucinates your conscious reality. https://www.ted.com/talks/anil_seth_your_brain_hallucinates_your_conscious_reality

Sharon Salzberg: https://www.sharonsalzberg.com/

Sims, R.E., Wu, H.H., & Dale, N. (2013). Sleep-wake sensitive mechanisms of adenosine release in the basal forebrain of rodents: An in vitro study. *PLoS One* 8(1):e53814.

Stanton, T.R., Moseley, G.L., Wong, A.Y.L., & Kawchuk, G.N. (2017). Feeling stiffness in the back: A protective perceptual inference in chronic back pain. *Sci Rep*. Aug 29;7(1):9681.

Steindl, S. (2020). *The Gifts of Compassion: How to Understand and Overcome Suffering*. Australian Academic Press.

Stephens, R., & Umland, C. (2011). Swearing as a response to pain – Effect of daily swearing frequency. *J Pain*. 12(12):1274–1281.

Stilwell, P., Harman, K. (2019). An enactive approach to pain: Beyond the biopsychosocial model. *Phenom Cogn Sci*. 18, 637–665.

Stulberg, B., & Magness, S. (2017). *Peak Performance: Elevate Your Game, Avoid Burnout, and Thrive with the New Science of Success*. Rodale Books.

Tamaki, M., Wang, Z., Barnes-Diana, T. et al. (2020). Complementary contributions of non-REM and REM sleep to visual learning. *Nat Neurosci.* 23:1150–1156.

Tara Brach. https://www.tarabrach.com/

Ten Percent app. https://www.tenpercent.com/

Thacker, M.A., & Moseley, G.L. (2012). First-person neuroscience and the understanding of pain. *Med J Aust.* Apr 2;196(6):410–411.

Thich Nhat Hanh. (2013). *The Art of Communicating*. Rider.

Thich Nhat Hanh. (2017). *The Art of Living*. Random House.

Thompson, E., & Varela, F. (2001). Radical embodiment: Neural dynamics and consciousness. *Trends Cogn Sci.* 5:418–425.

Tracey, I., & Mantyh, P.W. (2007). The cerebral signature for pain perception and its modulation. *Neuron.* Aug 2;55(3):377–391.

Tracey, K.J. (2021). From human to mouse and back offers hope for patients with fibromyalgia. *J Clin Invest.*131(13):e150382.

Tsakiris, M., & De Preester, H. (2019). *The Interoceptive Mind: From Homeostasis to Awareness*. OUP.

van der Kolk, B.A. (2014). *The Body Keeps the Score: Brain, Mind, and Body in the Healing of Trauma*. Viking.

Vannucci, A., Flannery, K.M., Ohannessian, & C.M. (2017). Social media use and anxiety in emerging adults. *J Affect Disord.* 1;207:163–166.

Varela, F., Thompson, E., Rosch, E. (2017). *The Embodied Mind: Cognitive Science and Human Experience*. The MIT Press.

Versus Arthritis. (2021). The state of musculoskeletal health 2021. Arthritis and other musculoskeletal conditions in numbers. https://www.versusarthritis.org/media/24238/state-of-msk-health-2021.pdf

Vlaeyan, J.W.S., & Linton, S.J. (2000). Fear-avoidance and its consequences in chronic musculoskeletal pain: A state of the art. *Pain* Apr;85(3):317–332.

Waking Up app: https://www.wakingup.com/

Walker, M. (2021). Matthew Walker's Defense of Napping: 5 Benefits of Napping. https://www.masterclass.com/articles/matthew-walkers-defense-of-napping

Wall, P.D. (1979). On the relation of injury to pain the John J. Bonica lecture. *Pain* Jun;6(3):253–264.

Walsh, B., Jamison, S., & Walsh, C. (2009). *The Score Takes Care of Itself: My Philosophy of Leadership*. Portfolio.

White, M.P., Alcock, I., Grellier, J. et al. (2019). Spending at least 120 minutes a week in nature is associated with good health and wellbeing. *Sci Rep.* 9:7730.

White, M.P., Elliott, L.R., Gascon, M., Roberts, B., & Fleming, L.E. (2020). Blue space, health and well-being: A narrative overview and synthesis of potential benefits. *Environ Res.* Dec;191:110169.

Witt, J.K., Linkenauger, S.A., Bakdash, J.Z., Augustyn, J.S., Cook, A., & Proffitt, D.R. (2009). The long road of pain: Chronic pain increases perceived distance. *Exp Brain Res.* 192(1):145–148.

Woods, H.C., & Scott, H. (2016). #Sleepyteens: Social media use in adolescence is associated with poor sleep quality, anxiety, depression and low self-esteem. *J Adolesc.* 51:41–49.

Yancey, P., & Brand, P. (1997). *The Gift of Pain: Why We Hurt and What We Can Do About It*. Zondervan.

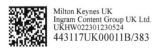

Milton Keynes UK
Ingram Content Group UK Ltd.
UKHW022301230524
443117UK00011B/383

9 781914 110283